TESTIMONIALS

Doctors like logic and science. This is a study plan which is logical and scientific, clear, concise, and unbelievably helpful. In Medicine one never stops learning. Prof. Tremayne's guide is not only helpful for exams but for lifelong learning and teaching.

Dr Charles Ovadia, MB, BS, FRACGP
(College Examiner)

I have accessed Patsy's expertise over the years for many of my surgical trainees and indeed for myself. Her approach in dealing with performance and anxiety under stressful conditions is exceptional. There is a lot to learn and no point in wasting time on poor study methods. I will be strongly recommending this book to all medical specialty trainees and medical students.

Dr Frank Piscioneri, FRACS, FRCS(Glas), MCh(Orth), MPH&TM
Supervisor of General Surgical Training
Clinical Director of Surgery
The Canberra Hospital, ACT

Patsy's approach to timing and planning study sessions for maximum efficiency cut my study sessions from 10hrs to 4hrs a day. More importantly, by providing a structured "pre-performance routine" for SAQs and viva stations, I approached the exam with confidence rather than trepidation. I wish I'd been taught how to study for exams in medical school.

Dr. Joanna Longley, FCICM, FACRRM, FRACGP
Staff Specialist, Hervey Bay Hospital, QLD.

Prof Patsy Tremayne has a background in sports psychology with extensive experience working with specialist trainees to enhance their exam performance, focussing on optimising learning practices, and improving communication skills and confidence. She is the key facilitator at the College of Intensive Care Medicine Written Exam Workshop and has been the guest speaker at several specialty exam courses, as well as providing one-on-one counselling sessions with trainees. In this way she has been helping trainees succeed in their specialist exams for more than twenty years. This book summarises her accumulated knowledge and experience, containing practical advice and tips on how to study smarter, not harder, with tried and tested study plans. This book is an invaluable resource for both trainees and their supervisors.

Dr. Mary Pinder, FCICM
Intensive Care Specialist, Sir Charles Gairdner Hospital, Perth
Chair, Assessments Committee, CICM
Vice-President, CICM

Passing exams has always been a difficult task for all of us, one which becomes easier over time; but sitting the Australian fellowship exams seems like a never-ending road – often leading to failure. Dear Patsy, you have the ability to not only show us a way to successfully passing these exams, you turned the whole journey into something fun: instead of feeling guilty every day, I did less studying but enjoyed it AND had time for myself - and passed the exams easily. You are a wonderful teacher – with this book you are going to help even more doctors to wear the gown at the fellowship ceremonies. There is nothing remotely similar – this book is unique, as is its brilliant writer!

Dr. med Nina Kloth, FANZCA
Fachaerztin fuer Anaesthesie & Notfall-und Gebirgsmedizin
Department of Anaesthesiology, Intensive Care - and Emergency Medicine
See-Spital Horgen & Kilchberg, Switzerland

ACE YOUR MEDICAL EXAMS

DR. PATSY TREMAYNE
PERFORMANCE PSYCHOLOGIST

Edited by Kath Walters.

Typset by Liz Seymour, Seymour Design.

Printed and bound by Ingram Sparks.

National Library of Australia Cataloguing-in-Publication entry

Title: Ace Your Medical Exams

Subtitle: Even when everything is stacked against you

ISBN: 978 0 6485482 0 1 (paperback)

Subjects: Psychology, communication, performance, education

It is a pleasure to be asked to contribute a few words for Dr Patsy Tremayne's book – a long awaited tome which I am sure will be much appreciated as a resource for medical practitioners starting along the path of vocational training examinations. Patsy has the unique ability to distil the extensive science surrounding learning and performing and provide practical, easily applicable strategies that make so much sense during a time of incredible stress. As a senior Intensive Care Specialist, I only wish I had known Patsy when I was training for my own specialist examinations. I will be putting this book straight onto the "must read" list for all our future specialist trainees!"

Dr Bronwyn Avard
(FCICM, MLMEd, PGCertCU, BMed)
(College Examiner)

I was absolutely delighted when Associate Professor Tremayne told me that she was writing a book to distil all her experience and knowledge in helping doctors and senior medical students pass their examinations. I have known about her work for many decades and have referred many young colleagues to her. I know of very few, if any, trainees who have not been helped to pass once they have had a few sessions with Patsy. I can particularly recall two contemporaries who had failed their College of Physicians clinical exams more than 5 times, usually coming croppers in their Short Cases. They had pretty well given up all hope. With Patsy's help they passed, and both are now highly respected Consultant Physicians.

In this fine book Patsy covers detailed approaches to all aspects of the study and examination tasks, and all bear repeated reading, thought and application. I commend it to the reader, and I fully expect it to take its place on the bookshelves of countless registrars and students, and the consultants responsible for their training and examination.

Professor John Watson AM
BSc (Hons I), MB, BS (Hons I), MD (Syd), DPhil (Oxon), FRACP, GAICD

For Connor, Will, and Sean
In the years to come

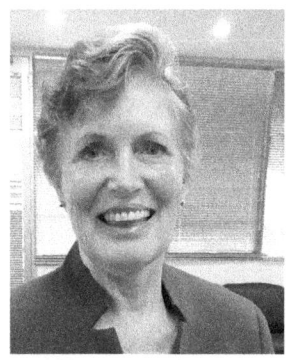

Dr. Patsy Tremayne is an Adjunct Associate Professor in the School of Social Sciences and Psychology at Western Sydney University, and was the first female sport and exercise psychologist in Australia. In 2007 she was awarded an Australian Psychological Society Award of Distinction for services to sport and exercise psychology.

Patsy has a private practice specifically focusing on performance enhancement for accredited medical trainees who need to study and pass major exams under often difficult and stressful conditions. She works with doctors all around Australia and New Zealand from all the major specialties. Her PhD in Psychophysiology from the University of NSW has been particularly useful in helping doctors to study smarter through the optimal use of the brain. The key is learning to practise under pressure to perform on demand.

ACKNOWLEDGEMENTS

I'm grateful to Sam Cawthorne for planting the seed regarding the writing of this book. He gently nagged me for such a long time, and I was very resistant. I'm also grateful for the willingness of my friends Colin Jones, to wade through the very first draft, and Annette Wallington-Jones for her encouragement over my inability to correctly use technology, and her wonderful skills with the use of Word.

I am indebted to busy members of the medical profession – Prof. Stuart Lane, for his kindness and incisive comments while reading chapters from the second draft, Dr. Andi Rauch, who made sure I knew the structure of the accreditation process for doctors in training schemes, and Dr. Rod Milton, who read the final draft. And, of course, I must thank Prof. Mohamed Khadra, who kindly offered to write the foreword.

For her professional help and encouraging words of wisdom I'd like to thank Kath Walters. She helped me put this book together and made my life a bit easier. I'd also like to thank Bernadette Foley for her editorial advice, Liz Seymour for her book designing and typesetting skills, Lu Sexton for her copy editing and skills as a wordsmith, and Peter Vaughan-Reid for such sharp eyes when proofreading.

My medical clients over the years have inspired me with their openness, honesty, and humour, in often trying situations. I would like to thank them each by name, but of course cannot. They generously shared themselves with me and provided material for this book.

It bothers me that I may have missed thanking some people, but whoever you are, you gave me the peace of mind that I needed to carry this project to completion.

FOREWORD

Dr Patsy Tremayne has been the reference for achieving high performance in medical examinations for over three decades now. I remember, as a young registrar in the early stages of my career, walking up the short pathway leading to her front door with trepidation. I was at the peak of my performance as a surgeon and was doubtful that a psychologist could possibly make me any better or even understand the intricacies of the examinations leading to the Fellowship of the Royal Australasian College of Surgeons. The same would be true of the various other Colleges of Medicine. How wrong I was. Within a couple of minutes, her abilities, insights and techniques became apparent. I realised that passing was not just about knowledge or skill but also, about technique, approach, mindfulness and motivations.

Since then, I have gone on to become a Senior Examiner for the College of Surgeons, a Professor of Surgery and Head of Clinical Surgery and continue to use her skills and approach in mentoring young registrars and candidates for the various examinations.

Her book, 'Ace Your medical Exams' is the synthesis and distillation of a lifetime of mentoring and assisting doctors on their way to specialty examinations and training. She presents material in a conversational way which at the same time is highly academic and based firmly in the literature on performance and adult study techniques.

I have, over the years, seen the fruits of Dr Tremayne's techniques through a number of younger colleagues who have benefitted from her sessions and time. I, and all of us involved in mentoring young doctors, thoroughly endorse this formalisation of her skills and approaches in this book.

Professor Mohamed Khadra AO
B Med, Grad Dip Comp, M Ed, PhD, FAICD, FRACS
Professor of Surgery University of Sydney

CONTENTS

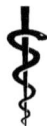

INTRODUCTION

"Medicine is a science of uncertainty, and an art of probability."

SIR WILLIAM OSLER

This book is all about how to study and have a structure, no matter what the challenges you face. I am going to give you a study structure that works even when you are under intense pressure with job commitments, having to do overtime and continual research, in addition to bringing up a family. You will regain control over the various aspects of life.

Doctors, if you read this book you will have an increased capacity to move forward, pass your exams more quickly and get on with life. You will feel more in control. Your career won't be on hold to quite the same extent. I believe by reading this book and following my system, you will increase self-awareness of your strengths and areas that need improvement.

I have created a system that uses the brain's optimal time to study and then later to perform and test various exam components under pressure. By practising regularly this regime becomes a habit.

There are three principles to this system:

1 **Content** – learning how to integrate, synthesise and remember the material; understanding the most appropriate times to study to optimise the use of the brain; using deliberate practice strategies to reinforce learning and develop good habits.

2 **Delivery** – learning how to get your message out there in oral and

written form. Exams are structured in a manner that tests the accuracy of responses under tight time conditions. This generates pressure. You will learn how to test your knowledge under speed-versus-accuracy conditions to enhance the speed and quality of your message.

3 **Perception** – learning about yourself and the art of engaging others. This involves several cognitive behavioural strategies and mindfulness techniques, such as adopting effective body language and using the voice in ways that engage the listener.

My private practice specifically focuses on performance enhancement for accredited medical trainees who need to study for major exams, often under difficult and stressful conditions. A typical medical trainee who would consult with me would be a senior registrar in a busy department of a major teaching hospital, let's say the Anaesthetic Department, perhaps in early to mid-thirties. Could be married and maybe has one or two young children. That person is also driven, anxious, and for the first time for years (or ever) is feeling incompetent. She or he has failed an exam!

This trainee has not failed before. They were one of the top students in high school and managed to get through every term in medical school without too much trouble. When applying for the anaesthetic training program they were often accepted at the first go – studied hard for the Primary exam and passed it. Now, three years later, they have failed the Fellowship exam. This is their first experience of failing an exam.

This person is constantly fatigued and quite fearful that they will fail again. They feel that there is nothing but studying and working all the time. They are losing physical fitness, they don't see the kids enough and feel guilty about it, and their partner is trying to hold down a job and look after the children as well. Their partner, although supportive, is certainly tired of bringing up the children virtually alone. Subconsciously, that partner may be adding to the pressure.

The trainee is still feeling ashamed and embarrassed about this failure, especially when others in the study group, who didn't do as well in the practice exams, seemed to pass with flying colours. This person has started to study again for the next exam sitting but feels disheartened and demotivated, with increasing procrastination and sabotaging thoughts. This is the sort of client I am dealing with all the time. This might be you.

The one thing most doctors tell me at their first visit, is that they just want to get their life back. They would like to have just a little bit of free time. Being in a specialist training program is a rigorous and gruelling process. One can spend up to 80 hours at work and still must find time to study on top of that. Any short breaks away, they take their study books. They long to pass their exams, get to see family and friends more often, relax and read some fiction when on holidays, and enjoy free time without the threat of constant study.

And what's coming up? Well, as you read, you will see my ideas are just a little bit different. I don't use jargon. I've obtained information from a variety of sources - from neuroscience to education, psychophysiology to sport psychology - and it's easy to read. There are questionnaires and action plans. There's information in there. There are stories you will identify with. (Names, specialties, gender and other details have all been changed or modified to maintain confidentiality of my clients, for whom I have the utmost admiration.)

WHO AM I, AND HOW CAN I HELP?

In summary, a little bit about me and why I think I'm the right person to write this book. Currently I'm an Adjunct Associate Professor in the School of Social Sciences and Psychology at Western Sydney University, in Sydney, New South Wales. My background is sport and exercise psychology, and in fact I was the first female sport psychologist to

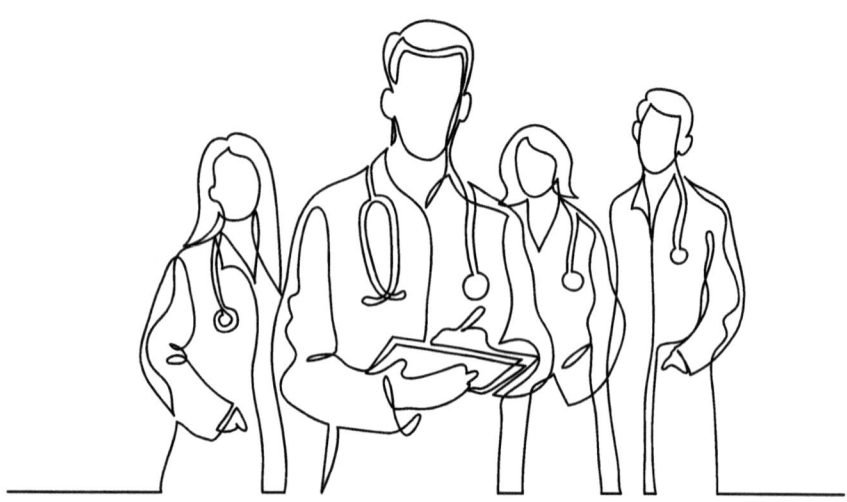

practise in Australia, way back in 1982. The university initiated a Masters in Sport Psychology Degree program in 1998, and I was director of this program till 2005. A couple of years later I was awarded an Australian Psychological Society Award of Distinction for services to sport and exercise psychology.

I still smile when I reflect on how I changed from having a thriving sport psychology practice to having a practice that focuses mostly on performance enhancement for accredited medical trainees. I was being interviewed about stress management on a Sydney radio program when a woman rang up and wanted my contact details. Her son had just failed his Fellowship exams for the second time. He was mortified and devastated.

The way he found out he had failed was particularly heart-breaking. A few hours after the oral exam trainees went to a list pinned up on a large wooden door. If their names were on the list, they had passed. They then opened the door, went inside and sipped champagne with the examiners. If their names were not on the list, they walked away, tail between their legs, feeling totally embarrassed and humiliated. This still happens with some colleges, but now exam candidates also have the choice to have their results emailed to them.

I worked for the next six to eight months with this doctor. I treated him like an athlete who has lost his motivation to train hard. I used many of the techniques I would use with athletes. I also had him describe to me in great detail all the components of each of the written and oral exams. I then worked out ways whereby he could practise these components under pressure. I also helped him plan meticulously for the exam days, just as I would with an athlete on competition days. I impatiently waited for the phone call to let me know if he had passed. He had. I was elated.

This was more exciting than getting an athlete onto an Australian team. From then on, I was hooked.

I work with doctors around Australia and New Zealand from all the major specialities. My PhD in psychophysiology from the University of New South Wales has been particularly useful in enabling me to help doctors to study smarter through the optimal use of the brain. The key to learning is to practise under pressure to perform on demand.

I also enjoy competing as a ballroom dancer in state and national events where the emphasis is on the artistry and athleticism of dance. And you know what? The intense focusing and refocusing that must take place for optimal performance in this sport helps my practice. Dancing is a wonderful way to practise and develop the same skills and strategies that I teach doctors as they prepare for their rigorous written and oral final exams.

A spiritual guru once said: "If you enjoy what you do then you never work a day in your life." And this is how I feel. I love what I do. I find helping doctors on their journey to get through their final exams is an honour and an amazing privilege. I have a front row seat and I see so many doctors go from being demoralised by failure to having an attitude of increased self-efficacy. Not fighting against the system but fighting and working with the system. And finally, getting through those challenging exams.

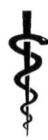

CHAPTER ONE

YOUR REALITY – LIFE AS A JUNIOR DOCTOR

"The difference between an adventure
and an ordeal is attitude."

BOB BITCHIN

Junior doctors have long reported struggling with mental health issues of overwork and exhaustion. At least two hospital departments in NSW had their training accreditation withdrawn in 2018 after complaints of bullying and harassment. You are carving out your career in a very tough environment. What you don't need, is to feel overwhelmed by study as well.

Most of the medical doctors who walk into my performance psychology practice complain about the dysfunctional training system they are in. Specifically, I am talking about the training system for junior doctors who must complete accredited programs as registrars to become specialist consultants.

If you are in this training system yourself, you will be aware how gruelling it is. For readers who may not be, I've summarised it below.

THE GRUELLING PATH TO BECOMING A SPECIALIST CONSULTANT

If a junior doctor who has just completed their first year as an intern wants to specialise in, for instance, neurosurgery, orthopaedics, emergency medicine, anaesthesia, or dermatology, in the following years as residents or senior resident medical officers they do four or five terms a year in different hospital departments. They usually have some choice for several of the terms during those years, and this is where doctors shape themselves into the direction they want to take. To become a specialist in a specific area of medicine they must apply to an accredited training program of a college. To be accepted for a training scheme of their choice, they must spend these early years gaining exposure to the skills of the specialty or sub-specialty they want to join. Then, when they are interviewed, they can show they already have some of the skills that are required.

Through references from consultants, through their CV, and then finally through an interview, they may get accepted into an accredited training program to do advanced training to become a specialist. They may need to travel interstate to take up that accredited program, as training positions can be limited. They may have a Primary/Part 1 exam in their initial years as a junior registrar/basic level trainee, and then it can take a further three or four years before they first sit their Fellowship/Part 2 exam at a senior registrar level. This is usually the final barrier to becoming a Fellow and then a consultant. As a registrar they often work with a variety of consultants, sometimes in different hospitals, with the emphasis on learning and practising in a variety of situations to round out training in their specialty. In some cases, the hospital's staff are unfriendly or unhelpful. Most of the consultants are competent and train their registrars well but, according to the anecdotes I hear. other consultants and staff bully and harass these doctors daily. This appears to happen quite regularly. The registrars report to me that they put up with this type of treatment, because it doesn't pay to "complain" or be

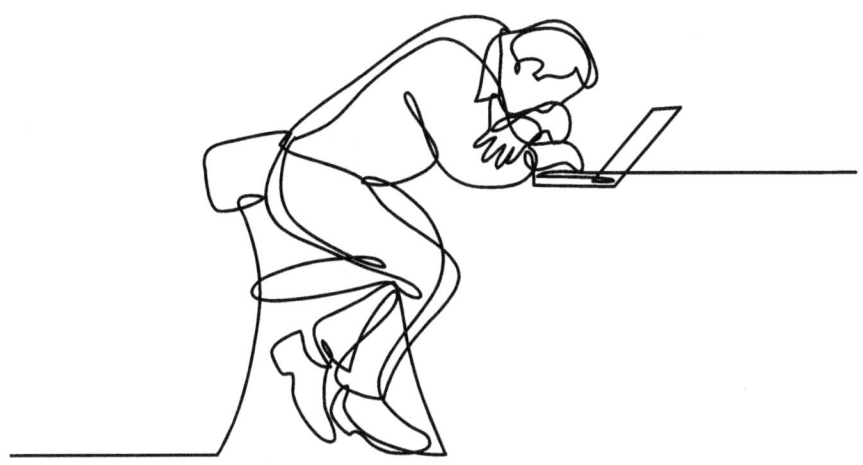

a "whistle-blower". It appears that some hospitals and individuals are much worse than others.

The impacts on family life are enormous. Doctors in training are so afraid of failure, they are too scared to complain. In fact, whistle-blowers do get punished. I had a client – a young surgeon – who was in a no-win situation. He had been sent interstate on a six-month rotation, but his final exam was during this rotation. He was attached to a consultant who was old-fashioned and did surgical techniques differently from the way this surgical trainee had been taught. And the consultant was grumpy. He was so grumpy that this trainee feared him. The trainee couldn't ask him questions and didn't think he could stay with this consultant until his exam. If the trainee complained about anything, or mentioned the way he'd been taught a technique, the consultant just said, "If you don't like it, get out of my theatre."

If the trainee had decided to complain to the college, it is likely the consultant would have been wrapped over the knuckles locally and he wouldn't have worked with the trainee anymore. But there was no other specialist in that city for the trainee to work with, so he wouldn't have finished his training in time for the exam. He would have had to spend another year in training. Even though it's not meant to be, it's a punishment for the whistle-blower. He must learn to keep his mouth shut, and just put up with the poor training and unpleasant environment.

You also have doctors who are growing up without seeing their kids. One trainee I worked with was posted to Canberra for six months while her two children, aged two and three years-old stayed with their father in Sydney. She had to do this posting. She came up whenever she got time off: every two weeks. Another male doctor was posted to another city to complete his training. He saw his five year-old girl and his wife about once a month.

All this contributes to these doctors failing the required exams to become specialists. These failing doctors are normally high-performing individuals, who've passed all their high school exams, and all their medical training to be doctors. They may not have failed previously in their lives. And suddenly, they are failing.

THE EFFECTS OF FAILING A FELLOWSHIP EXAM

When doctors fail, they begin to feel incompetent. Isolation and humiliation accompany their failure and it gets worse as they face the possibility of failing for a second, third or fourth time. Consequently, their training may take even longer than three or four years. Every time they sit these exams, they must pay a fee of thousands of dollars. The fee set depends on the college. When these doctors make an appointment to see me, they are often at the end of their tether, feeling out of control and desperate. Sometimes, they're on the verge of tears. My clients are often just at the age where they are having young kids. This intense pressure means they feel they're overwhelmed and don't have enough time to study.

Many of the trainees I see are from overseas and English may be a second language. There may be cultural differences that need to be considered, and their extended family may not be in Australia, which can lead to isolation and loneliness. Overall, there may be extra pressure and a lack of institutional and family support that is not experienced to the same extent by locally trained candidates.

This book will give you a structure and a plan, which will enable you to regain control.

PSYCHOLOGICAL DISTRESS

A survey on thousands of doctors and medical students in 2013 by *beyondblue* showed the extent of psychological distress experienced by this group of workers. According to former chairman the Hon. Jeff Kennett AC, the findings revealed the extent of doctors' and medical students' suffering and should act as an immediate rallying call for action. He said: "This survey builds on our previous work in this area and we hope it also serves as a wake-up call to the Australian medical community that more must be done to tackle things such as over-work and discriminatory attitudes."

In early 2019, newspapers reported on a trainee who was hospitalised for sleep deprivation after working up to 24 consecutive days on-call at a Sydney hospital. This brought to national attention the possible exploitation of medical trainees regarding on-call work and un-rostered overtime which was not claimed.

From time to time, I see newspaper articles about doctors who have committed suicide. Some of those people sadly are, just like my clients, doctors in training to become specialists. To be honest, I've had people in my office I have been worried about because they feel so desperate and are certain they're not going to pass their exams.

If this sounds like you, this book is about putting you back in control. Maybe you are not a doctor, but a university or high school student. That is fine because these techniques will work for you too.

YOU ARE NOT ALONE

You are not alone if you are struggling to manage the pressure of study. It is a widespread problem among doctors. For many years I have worked almost exclusively in my practice with doctors. Through word of mouth, my practice changed over time from working with athletes and performing artists to primarily working with doctors throughout Australia and New Zealand. As an accredited psychologist, and a former academic, I've become an authority in this area.

Here's how I define "authority": It's who you are as a person, your character, the influence you've built in your field over many years. It's familiarity with relevant research, perhaps in neuroscience, psychophysiology, education, or sport and exercise dealing with performance. I'm familiar with the research in my area and can usually find appropriate material whenever I need it.

In my first career, I was an elite athlete. I was a high-board diver, and I trained mostly in the United States. I made it to the Commonwealth Games and got a third place representing Australia. But I was always scared of heights, and I realised I needed much more than physical fitness to succeed. I needed to control fear. So, I then thought, "Gee, I'd like to be a psychologist." I decided, with my sporting background, to become a sport psychologist. There were no training programs in Australia at the time, so I went to the United States, and did a postgraduate degree in Sport Psychology. I came back to Australia and did a PhD in psychophysiology which is physiology and psychology: the study of body and mind. Then I started working with my first medical clients and I realised I loved working with doctors more than with athletes, so now I work almost exclusively in this field.

However, there are many, many sad stories. I would like that culture to change, and it can. We are facing generational change; these young doctors going through can be the ones who make that change happen.

ARE YOU OVERWHELMED?

When I write blogs about these cases, I get calls from people saying, "You're talking about me. That's me!" They recognise the symptoms. One of the chronic symptoms is performance anxiety. Performance anxiety can mean that, as the exam comes closer, you think only of failing. Your stomach churns, your knees go weak, you start to feel a bit sick. You find you can't concentrate on what you are doing; and this gets worse as time goes by. If you have already failed once or twice, these symptoms can be exacerbated. You might notice this performance anxiety leads to diminishing confidence and perceived incompetence. You feel, "I'm not good enough, I'm not going to pass". You might find you are not being assertive enough to ask for time off or better shifts closer to exams. Of course, you must be careful not to be disrespectful as there is a strong hierarchy in medicine, and consultants and hospital administrators do wield power.

Sometimes, a client will complain that they are not getting proper training. For instance, I often get doctors who have failed once or twice in their exams. They're then put onto rotations that might be in regional hospitals. Perhaps they are rostered to do lots of night shifts. Sometimes there is no consultant at the regional hospital, and if there is, they are certainly not working at night. They don't work nights unless they get called out for an emergency. So, the doctor in training is deemed competent enough to work nights, but there's no consultant available to train them. This means that the trainee isn't getting enough training in different procedures because they're being used as a workhorse in the regional hospital. They are doing it competently, but they're not training towards their exam. So, sometimes they try to go to other hospitals in their own time, and beg consultants to give them vivas, or allow them to observe different procedures. Perhaps they take on extra work doing locums in private hospitals.

There is a particularly sad story of a female surgical trainee who was sitting her Fellowship exam for the second time. She worked full-time and did shift work too. She had a stay-at-home husband. They had three children who were supposed to be looked after by the husband when they came home after school. However, her husband virtually ignored them. But he kept saying to his wife that he could cope, and he didn't need an au pair or help with the housework, or somebody to mind the children. So, the wife did almost everything.

She was totally exhausted. When she was at home and trying to study, her husband didn't keep control of the children, so they were knocking on her door the whole time. They, of course, wanted to see her and spend time with her. She was not able to study efficiently. She had no time. So, she had performance anxiety on top of the exhaustion. And she was guilty about not seeing her children enough.

INTERNAL STRESSES ARE AS BAD AS EXTERNAL ONES

Not all stories are as sad as this one. Some trainees don't have these kinds of stresses. They have very supportive partners, or they don't have children, or they live alone, or have good rotations where the hospital departments are helpful, and the consultants are kind and train people well. Maybe they have reasonable shifts because there is a good supply of registrars at that hospital.

For these people, their problems may well be internal, rather than related to the environment. It could be they procrastinate; maybe they've always been procrastinators. Sometimes they have a lack of motivation; they've failed once or twice, and they are bored just doing the same old study again. I often find most people who failed their exams two or three times have the knowledge, but don't know how to study smartly.

In some instances, I get people ringing me in January when they have an upcoming exam that's in February or March. They say, "Okay, I'm about to take time off and I'm going to study 12 hours a day!" I try to persuade these trainees that cramming at the last minute isn't great; but that's what they've done previously for the HSC or in med school, and it worked. However, it just doesn't often work in these exams, and trainees usually find that out.

It's better to chip away at study and testing over time.

Of course, some people do get through their exams more easily. Perhaps they get through because their hospital terms are a bit easier, and they have helpful consultants. Believe me, there are some very good, helpful consultants who really try to get their trainees through the exam process.

But I know that if you have picked up this book, it is because you are among the many students who are struggling and need help. My clients all need some help to organise their study or prepare for interviews. My insights, gathered from my work with doctors over decades, can help you regardless of whether you are a doctor, or whether you are a university student or a high school student, or you just need to study smarter.

ASK YOURSELF THESE QUESTIONS BEFORE YOU TURN THE PAGE

Be honest with yourself before you answer this quiz. Reflect on how effective you think your study technique is today. There are techniques in the following chapters that teach you how to overcome procrastination, sabotaging thoughts, and distractions. There are evidence-based study hints to help you maintain control and chip away at the overwhelming amount of work required to pass your exams. Change is scary, but I'm sure you've identified with some of the problems discussed in this chapter. Circle a score from 1 (not likely) to 10 (most likely) for each question.

QUESTION #1
Would I improve my study techniques if I used this guide?

1	2	3	4	5	6	7	8	9	10

NOT LIKELY   MAYBE   MOST LIKELY

QUESTION #2
Would my confidence improve if these hints worked for me?

1	2	3	4	5	6	7	8	9	10

NOT LIKELY   MAYBE   MOST LIKELY

QUESTION #3
Would my performance anxiety decrease if I followed this program?

1	2	3	4	5	6	7	8	9	10

NOT LIKELY   MAYBE   MOST LIKELY

QUESTION #4

Could I honestly change what I do now?

1	2	3	4	5	6	7	8	9	10

NOT LIKELY   MAYBE   MOST LIKELY

QUESTION #5

Could I start off with small changes?

1	2	3	4	5	6	7	8	9	10

NOT LIKELY   MAYBE   MOST LIKELY

QUESTION #6

Will I start using the techniques in this guide this week?

1	2	3	4	5	6	7	8	9	10

NOT LIKELY   MAYBE   MOST LIKELY

QUESTION #7

Now that I've read this far, could it be fear that says, "I haven't got time" or "It's safer to continue as I am"?

1	2	3	4	5	6	7	8	9	10

NOT LIKELY   MAYBE   MOST LIKELY

These questions give an indication as to where you are on the Stages of Change (see Chapter 8 for more details).

Above 55: You're ready for action according to the Stages of Change (Prochaska & DiClemente, 1983).

40 to 54: You're just a little more cautious and are still in the preparation stage.

21 to 39: You may be in the contemplation stage.

20 or less: You may be in the pre-contemplation stage of change. However, you may well find that reading further chapters may motivate a desire to change.

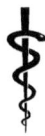

CHAPTER TWO

STRUCTURE IS THE SECRET TO SMART STUDY

"Failure is normal in an ambitious life."

ANON.

A structure is the linchpin of the system in this book. Having a plan of study that is well structured is going to help you feel less overwhelmed. You will use your brain wisely, feel more in control, and have more time to spend with family and friends. You will have a sense of confidence, rather than dread, at the thought of the upcoming exams. You're much more likely do better in these exams than you've ever done before by using these techniques. I've seen this system work many times.

Most medical students approach study in a very ad hoc way. They try to find the time, squeezing it in where they can without considering whether it is the optimal time to study. Of course, not everything you are doing is wrong. Whether you are a doctor or a university student, you are here because you are good at what you do. You are good at studying. You got through high school with top marks. You got into medical school or university without failing. It's only now, when you're under a great deal of pressure, that you need to handle the exams differently. You can't cram for these exams. You need to chip away. There is so much information to learn. Now, you need to have a much more coordinated approach to the way you study.

WHY DOES STRUCTURE MATTER?

A structured approach to your study prevents you from feeling overwhelmed. You stop feeling that you are not doing enough, that you haven't got the time. You'll be in a better place and feel better. When you feel happier, you have a greater possibility of passing your exams and passing them well.

A structure is like a building's foundations. If it's strong and if you can put down building blocks of the basic structure, then it's likely to work better for you. It is stable.

DON'T PUT YOUR LIFE ON HOLD

I set up a program for a young surgical trainee. She was really pleased to have a study plan, and when she came back the second time, she had done everything I had asked of her. However, she said she was very tired. I had thought that I could add one more item to her study. I was going to get her to do one short answer question for only 10 minutes a night after she came back from work. She looked at me, and she said, "I'll try, but I think I'm way too tired. I'm too hungry." That made the hairs on the back of my neck prickle. What have I missed here?

I said, "You're hungry? What does that mean?"

"Well, I haven't eaten all day," she said.

"Well, when did you last eat?"

"Oh, I ate last night."

"Last night? Twenty-four hours ago?"

"Yes. I only eat once a day. I haven't got time."

"Why haven't you got time?"

"Well, I'm in the theatre sometimes from 7.30 am right up to 8 pm."

"What time do you get up?" I asked.

"I get up at 7 am because I don't get to bed until late. I have a quick cup of coffee as I rush out the door to get my Uber to work."

"Why don't you have a bunch of bananas just sitting there so you can grab one and perhaps eat it in the Uber on the way to work."

"Yeah, I didn't think of that," she said. "But I don't like to eat in front of the Uber driver."

"Offer the driver a banana if you like. Don't worry about that!"

This exchange shocked me. Here was this very bright registrar who wasn't giving any thought to the fact that her body and brain were not working well. She was exhausted because she wasn't eating. She wasn't looking after herself. It didn't occur to her that she could have a nutritious snack on the run.

Also, it is more than just not eating. Perhaps you never take a break and you feel exhausted. I often see medical trainees who feel very down because they're not spending quality time with their partners or their families. Maybe the kids want to see them more of them. Maybe the partner is pressuring them, saying, "Look, you've got to pass your exams next time. We can't go on like this."

Is this you? Perhaps you are distracted by the demands at the hospital; you're often tired and very tense when you come home. You're often unable to get to sleep, or you toss and turn in the night. Maybe you're studying right up until bedtime. You're eating badly. You're not seeing your friends; you're not going out for coffees; you're not doing the usual things that ordinary people do.

What I see is chaos, and what I will do in this book is give you structure. I will provide a little structure to reduce the confusion, and you hang on to that. Then you will see that you're chipping away at some study. It's not all work and overtime.

Let me ask you: How often do you study after work? You come home after a 12 to 14-hour day. Perhaps you bathe the kids if you have them. Or you might sit down, have a quick snack, and then sit at your desk from 8 pm until 10 pm or even 12 am. You go to bed, and you get up at 5 am, ready to start at 6 or 7 or 8 am. Much of the information you studied the previous night is gone. After a long day at work, it is not going into your long-term memory.

Or maybe you think, "I'm too tired. I can't do this." Well, I don't blame you. Young doctors (aged 30 and under) work the longest hours of any age group: 49.8 hours a week compared to a mean of 43.6, according to statistics from a *beyondblue* survey. No wonder you are tired. This is another reason to have some structure.

Or maybe you procrastinate. You can tell if you're a procrastinator if you do the following:

1. Overestimate how much time you have left to perform tasks.
2. Underestimate how long it takes to complete tasks.
3. Tell yourself you will feel motivated tomorrow, or after you've had a good night's sleep, or similar.
4. Think that you need to feel like studying in order to remember it well.
5. Believe that studying when not in the mood isn't going to work.

It can get even worse than that. Occasionally, doctors turn to drugs or alcohol. In fact, in a survey by *beyondblue* in 2013 the mean percentage of doctors by specialty who drink at high risk or harmful levels is 2.5 per cent. I had a surgical trainee a few years ago who hadn't turned up at work. She hadn't been performing well and her bosses feared suicide. When the police went around to her apartment, they found her at home with empty alcohol bottles everywhere.

That's an extreme example, but more common than we realise. My clients don't often talk to me about their alcohol or drug problems because that's not what they've come to see me for. I'm not in the business of treating these problems. I'm trying to provide them with a better study structure so that they don't feel tempted to use drugs or alcohol for comfort or release.

GET PAST THE BARRIERS

You have a barrier hampering your ability to move ahead and to get on with your career. That barrier is your exams, so your life seems to be on hold.

The problems you face affect other people, too. Your family's life is also on hold. Your partner, whoever's in the supporting role, is looking after the kids and waiting for you to pass your exams. Sometimes you and your partner are both sitting exams, and if you have children this is

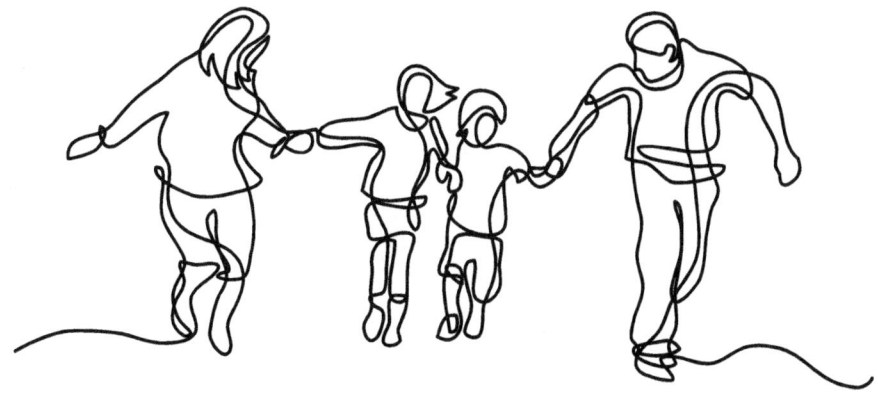

especially difficult for everyone. But if you have a plan, a structure, then you feel more in control.

One doctor came up to me after I'd given a lecture and told me he just wasn't able to concentrate on his study any more. When I asked him why, he said he just couldn't help thinking about his 12-month old baby boy who was growing up without him. He told me he left too early in the morning to see him, and when he came home he had so much study to do that he only briefly hugged him and kissed him goodnight. I suggested to him that he would study better if he allocated half an hour each evening to play with the child; that this would enable him to study more efficiently. I felt that he was grieving because he wasn't seeing his little boy enough. He rang me a few weeks later and said that things were a lot better.

ARE YOUR EMOTIONS CONTROLLING YOU?

QUESTION #1

Do your eyes prick with tears during moving scenes in books or films?

A	No, not at all	Score	a = 1
B	Sometimes	Score	b = 3
C	Quite often	Score	c = 5

QUESTION #2

If your partner was flirting with someone else at a party, would you:

A	Feel pretty bad about it, but you wouldn't show it?	Score	a = 3
B	Take no notice?	Score	b = 1
C	Go home in a huff?	Score	c = 5

QUESTION #3

There is no one else at home and you are reading in bed.
You hear a strange noise. What would your very first thought be?

A	It's only a cat	Score	a = 1
B	Someone is breaking in	Score	b = 3
C	The place is haunted	Score	c = 5

QUESTION #4

How often do you really lose your temper?

A	Very seldom	Score	a = 1
B	Sometimes	Score	b = 3
C	Quite a lot	Score	c = 5

(Adapted from W. Morgan & P. Tremayne, 1985)

Questions 1 to 4 give an indication as to the way your emotions control you. If your score for these four questions is:

16 or more: Your emotions are on a see-saw. If you're happy, it shows in your demeanour, and when you're feeling down, everyone knows it. Keep in mind that emotions are short-lived, and resist impulsive actions. A better study structure may help stabilise your emotions.

10 to 15: It's not that you don't feel things, but you control your emotions fairly well, so others aren't always aware of how you feel. Be aware that you will get support from colleagues and friends if you express any doubts and fears.

9 or less: You don't really show your emotions much. Others may see you as being a bit cold blooded, but you see yourself as being practical and logical. This can stand you in good stead, especially if you're in a department which has an unfriendly culture.

Don't take this do-it-yourself test too seriously. Use it as a guide. It might point you in the right direction and give you more self-awareness. You may recognise that your emotional state is influenced by not having a good study structure which includes rest breaks.

Most students are not experts in studying; they're medical experts or experts in other fields. There's a lot of information about studying out there, and it's hard to tell what works. There are lots of available study programs. There are many well-meaning doctors who will give you advice, but it's usually not evidence-based. Instead, it is anecdotal: "I did this and I got through, so why don't you try it?"

When it gets close to the Higher School Certificate, I look at all the different strategies that students say they use. And the ones that resonate with me are the students who say, "I take some time off. I get out. I don't study all day." In fact, taking a break and having a rest is one of the most important parts of my structure. I am going to address that in the next chapter.

You will see that this book is about acing your exams AND having a life. You don't have to put your life on hold. I read a lot of research papers and material around studying at optimal times for the brain. Based on my reading, working with my clients and getting their valuable feedback, I know I'm on the right track.

This is my structured study program in a nutshell, and it is all based on what the brain needs.

First, you need to recover from the system you're now using.

If you are reading this book, you're either at the end of your tether or you're looking for some other way to optimise your study. You need to heal.

Next, I'll show you how to pay attention: how to increase your attentional focus, and when the best times are to focus attention.

Then, you need some cognitive behavioural and mindfulness approaches that are going to help you use your energy wisely.

I'll show you how to test yourself under pressure so that you can replicate dealing with the stress during written and clinical exams.

After regular practice, when all this becomes a habit, you won't have so many of those self-sabotaging thoughts. During clinical exams, the emphasis needs to be on the ability to communicate your message clearly. That communication needs to be both verbal and nonverbal to engage your listeners, the examiners.

Finally, I look at self-confidence and how to recognise that, yes, this is working. People are complimenting you. You're thinking, "I've changed. I'm working better, and I feel better than before I adopted this structured approach."

HAVE TIME ON YOUR SIDE

Sometimes people come to me and say, "I've got my exam in six weeks." Well, my study system takes time to implement. It takes time to develop good study habits. The earlier you start, the better you will get at it. But if you've left your run late, you can still benefit from the strategies in this this book. As soon as you get started, things will get better. The further you go, the better it will be.

I've carefully planned the order of the tasks I give you. Given enough time, up to the exam, you can use the structure, and use it wisely. Your friends, family, partner, and kids will be happier, and so will you.

Simplicity is the key. This structured plan is easy to understand (study in the morning, test yourself after work). It's easy to follow and has enough wiggle room to allow for changes and unexpected obstacles.

Ask yourself the following questions, and circle a score from 1 to 10 for each question.

QUESTION #1

How structured do you think your study is at the moment?

1	2	3	4	5	6	7	8	9	10

NOT STRUCTURED   STRUCTURED

What kinds of distractions make that structure crumble: the kids getting sick, the car needing a service, an additional shift, or your partner getting upset?

QUESTION #2

How effective is your current study structure?

1	2	3	4	5	6	7	8	9	10

NOT EFFECTIVE   EFFECTIVE

Has this chapter changed your view of structure? Can you see how a structure like this might work? Are you open to the idea of bringing a new structure into your study?

Well, if you know that it is time to test a new structure, then I'd like to start with one of my most popular ideas: recovery.

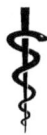

CHAPTER THREE

RECOVERY COMES FIRST

"It's OK to not be OK, as long as you don't stay that way."

ANON.

There are three basic principles in my study system. The first is to learn about yourself and your needs, and how to recover, which is what we will cover in this chapter. The brain works optimally if you can achieve a better life-work balance. You will have better mental, physical and emotional health. This can be achieved by changing from your long, ineffective study hours, and recovering by working smarter, not harder.

When clients come to see me, they're often at the end of the road. They feel exhausted and overwhelmed. You cannot be effective with a new study routine when you feel this way. You can start it, but you must have time to recover.

Recovery is important. A brain that has been stressed and overworked for an extended period cannot think clearly.

So, improve your physical, mental and emotional health first.

You'll find that you work better and do better quality study by doing less. You have used your brain during hours that are not optimal for learning. Subconsciously, you are aware that you cannot take in as much as you should. You have not retained what you learned. If you have a partner, they are over it, especially if this is your second or third attempt. They want to get on with life, perhaps they want to start a family, and everything is on hold until you pass that exam.

After I explain to my clients how the brain works, I tell them to spend some time with their friends and family and to not go near their desk during the afternoons of their days off. They break into a grin and say, "Oh, I can do that." Then I give them their study hours, and they say, "This is so much less than I've been doing."

INVEST THE TIME TO RECOVER

Sometimes, students say, "Are you sure? Is this enough? Am I doing enough?" It's a good question. If you have failed twice or more in this exam, then I believe you know your material. What you don't have is the ability to retain it and manage the pressure of the exams. However, if you have not sat the exam before then I don't know how much knowledge you have under your belt. Here's what I recommend: Start off by studying less. Let yourself recover first, and if you need to do more, we'll add to your schedule later.

Ahead, we are going to look at how to recover your physical, mental and emotional health.

Under physical health, we will look at nutrition and exercise, circadian rhythms and how to use the brain to remember and integrate material at the right time. We will also look at how you can rest and recuperate and have good sleep hygiene, so you get quality sleep at night.

Under mental health, we will look at how to use your brain wisely, knowing when to study and when to take a break. This helps your wellbeing quite a bit. A lot of doctors I see come from other countries, which have different training systems and different cultures, where teachers are highly respected and always right. These trainees are humble and taught at young ages not to argue or disagree with their superiors. Sometimes, these doctors are bullied. So, we will look at how to stand up a little bit and respectfully say, "No, I think somebody else deserves to work some of this overtime and not me all the time."

As far as your emotional health is concerned, we will have a look at your priorities. If it makes you happy to spend more time with friends or family or kids, I build this into your structure, so you can spend time away from your desk feeling guilt-free. Better work-life balance leads to enhanced emotional resilience. You are going to feel a lot better.

THESE ARE LIFE SKILLS THAT WILL SERVE YOU THROUGHOUT YOUR CAREER

When you're happier, you're more relaxed, and your brain is working more effectively. The chances are, you get improved results in both your clinical vivas and in the written exams. I can't guarantee you'll pass these exams, but I bet you'll do better than you've done before.

If you adopt this structure and use it daily, it becomes a habit. You don't even think about it. You won't procrastinate as much. These are techniques that are useful throughout life. Teach them to your kids, and to your partner. And down the track they'll be helpful in your consultancy.

Be open to these new ideas. If you want to change, try what I suggest and see what happens. You are going to need a few tools. Here's a list:

- A smartphone with a recording device, ready for when consultants question you. With the consultant's permission, record your responses and the feedback that the consultant gives you. Then you don't need to think about it again during the day. Take the pressure off and listen to the recording at your leisure.

- A small paper diary so that you can monitor your progress. It must be a paper diary. Evidence shows that if you write rather than type, you remember more.

- A digital kitchen timer. A digital timer is more accurate to time all the tasks I will talk about later in this book. It's just as important to stop on time to as it is to start on time.

- Noise cancelling headphones for studying at home, particularly if you have young children.

- An interval timer. This is like a pedometer – it can be clipped onto the inside of your underpants. You can set it for specific times to vibrate. This is useful as a reminder for various tasks I will give you. It can be worn in theatre when you're scrubbed up and cannot use other devices. Some fitbits and smart watches include an interval timing device.

STUDYING FROM HOME: A CASE STUDY

I remember my first consultation with Jane. She preferred to study upstairs in her bedroom, but she couldn't because she had two young children who, if they knew she was in the house, would be often clamouring for her. So, she would spend about 40 minutes travelling to and from the local library to get some peace. She would wave goodbye to the children and off she would go. The kids would happily go back inside with their father and play. I said, "No! You're wasting 40 minutes each day going to and from the library. We need to find a way so that you can work in your bedroom." Here's what she did.

Whenever she wanted to study at home, she'd go to the front door with the kids, and she'd wave goodbye as usual. She'd walk down the path and close the gate. Their father would take the kids into the living room and play with them. She'd sneak up the side of the house, in the back door, and creep up the stairs to her room. Then she'd put on her noise cancelling headphones and get to work. She found that she was able to do good quality study, and she had valuable extra free time in each day.

REFLECT ON YOUR LIFESTYLE AND CIRCUMSTANCES NOW

If you reflect on what's happening in your environment, in your situation, it's going to increase self-awareness. You can't change unless you have self-awareness. You must understand how failure and work have affected you. Because, under stress, you lose sight of your priorities. You think the only solution is to work harder. People who have failed once usually decide they must study more to pass. The second time, the third time, study more, study more. It gets harder to become motivated to study. They see even less of their family. They become doctors who work, study, and do nothing much else.

Set aside a little time. Just sit in the sun, enjoy a break, and reflect on your situation. Often, when people come to see me, it is the first time they have thought about what is going on in their life. I used to see a very busy dermatology trainee. She had clinical meetings every night, and very little time to study. As soon as she walked into my office, she burst into tears. So, I said, "Look, you've got to sit down and think about where you are, what you're doing and let's work on ways you can change." By the time she came back to the second session, she had given it some thought and was ready to make some changes.

HOW SELF-ASSURED ARE YOU?

QUESTION #1

When nothing seems to be going right for you, do you usually:

A Analyse how much of it is your own fault?	Score	a = 1
B Put the blame on someone else?	Score	b = 5
C Shrug your shoulders – it was just bad luck?	Score	c = 3

QUESTION #2

Do you like being the centre of attention?

A Sometimes – depends on how I feel	Score	a = 3
B Certainly	Score	b = 5
C No, I don't	Score	c = 1

QUESTION #3

When you have to make a decision about something, do you?

A Ask around and see what other people think?	Score	a = 1
B Reach a quick decision that may or may not be right?	Score	b = 5
C Give yourself time and go over all the angles?	Score	c = 3

QUESTION #4

If you ever do lie, is it often because:

A You don't want to step on someone's toes?	Score	a = 3
B You want to create a good impression?	Score	b = 5
C You are nervous or embarrassed?	Score	c = 1

Questions 1 to 4 tell you how secure you feel in the world around you. If your score for these totals is:

16 or more: You are fairly confident and secure. You have a dominant personality and you really like your own way. Keep this in mind while you're a trainee in the hierarchical world of medicine and think before you 'rock the boat'.

9 or less: You're a bit of a worrier, and don't always feel too secure. You like to be organised and know what's going on, to minimise your worrying thoughts.

10 to 15: You're confident and sure of yourself, but not overbearing. Nor do you worry too much. You see harassment and negative comments for what they are and handle yourself well.

DETERMINE YOUR PRIORITIES

Doing this will make you more amenable to prioritising your time. Most people understand this when they have some time to think it over. Once your priorities are sorted out, then managing your time becomes simpler. Understand what you must do for your physical, emotional and mental wellbeing first. Everyone can do this, but some people have difficulty. If that is you, find someone who can help you reflect by asking you questions. It's something I do with my clients; ask questions that help them to reflect.

Sometimes people have problems other than exams and priorities. You might have sick or dependent relatives. In some instances, I recommend that you see somebody else to sort out other clinical issues you may have. If you have moderate to severe depression or generalised anxiety, you may need more support from other services.

Once you know what matters to you,
it is easier to cut out the procrastination.

If you organise family time in the afternoon, you know you must balance that with your study in the morning. You will find that you have better quality study. The family leave you alone to do your work because they know they will see you later in the afternoon. I strongly suggest that you have recreation in the afternoon. See your children, or go shopping, or catch up with friends. Avoid sitting at that desk and studying.

One obstetrics and gynaecology trainee I worked with had days off during the week. After she worked out what was important for her, she made arrangements that others would take the children to day care. She then could study in the morning and would be free to pick them up in the afternoon.

SUCCESS STORY

An anaesthetic registrar came to me after she'd been doing the study program for a few weeks, and said, "This plan works. I'm studying in the morning. My partner was complaining to me all the time, saying, 'You spend all day studying! I never get time to see you.' Now, he knows that I finish at midday. We went out and had lunch with friends the other day. I feel so much better now that I've changed." This registrar felt more in control.

You cannot manage your time unless you know what your priorities are. Sometimes it's tough to know what your priorities are, isn't it? You can be pulled every which way. If you have a sick relative or child, they need immediate attention. It happens. All you can do is just snatch time when you can to study in the morning and rest in the afternoon. Then get back to the routine as soon as you can.

MANAGE YOUR TIME: HOW AND WHEN TO STUDY (AND WHY)

Time management means that if you say you are going to do something at a specific time, you do it. You've made a promise to yourself. Time management means sticking to those commitments. Often there are times when other engagements look more attractive, but you must ask yourself, "Is study the top priority for you?" If it is, then sit down to study at eight o'clock on a Saturday morning, and keep going till midday. You know that that's the time you've set aside so you adjust times for other engagements.

When you study in the morning, you've got an activating prefrontal cortex. It helps you to integrate and synthesise material better.

> You will place the material you read more readily into long-term memory when the brain is rested.

Make it a rule to study in the morning on your days off. That time is precious. Turn your phone and other notifications off. Don't look at your emails. Make that your study time. Then you can do what you like in the afternoon. That's the reward.

SUCCESS STORY

A urology registrar had complained to me that he couldn't remember stuff, despite studying all day every free weekend. He was quite miserable and very tired. Over time, as he started to study in the morning only, he noticed that he recalled facts more readily when he tested himself. He was quite cheered up by that. He said, "It's like my brain seems to be working again."

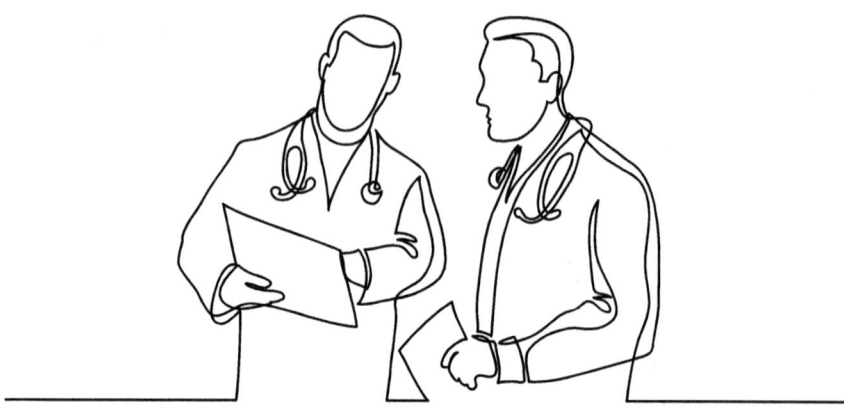

LEARN THE ART OF RESPECTFUL ASSERTIVENESS

Sometimes, if your superiors ask you to work more hours, do you find that you can't refuse? Maybe you are one of three registrars studying together during a short break. When the roster supervisor comes in, they ask the person they know is more likely to say yes, because it's easier. That person could be you, even though somebody else may not have had a weekend roster for weeks. It's unfair sometimes. You don't want to be the one who gets all the weekend rosters. You do need to learn how to say no respectfully. You can't possibly manage your own time if you cannot make a commitment and assert yourself. If you are a bit shy, it takes a little bit longer to become assertive. But when you commit to managing your time, you realise the value of doing so.

Here's what you might respectfully say when you turn down a shift, "No thank you. I have other commitments. I've been doing it for three weekends in a row. I think it's somebody else's turn." You know what? The supervisory staff may end up having a bit more respect for you. You might think you're being polite when you accept all the shifts; they might think you're a doormat. When you have a voice, they take you into account. You're just subtly reminding them to be a bit fairer.

Sometimes asserting yourself in front of other people might cause problems, so organise an appointment with your supervisor or with the person doing the rosters. Point out any perceived unfairness in the rosters and ask if you could have a weekend off.

Ali was an emergency medical registrar. He told me it was inevitably him who was asked to do overtime on public holidays. He said, "I'd be in a room with other registrars, all sitting there studying for our exams. The person doing the rosters would always ask me first. I didn't like to refuse." I encouraged Ali to learn to say no. He was very shy about it and didn't want to do it, but in the end, he did. He found the selection process a bit fairer from then on.

As a doctor, there are times when you must be assertive. It's an important skill to learn. And in this context, by being assertive, you're giving yourself a chance to study at times that suit your brain. You give your brain a rest at times when it needs to recuperate. You use the times when your circadian rhythms allow you to study thoroughly.

GIVE THAT BRAIN A REST – USE YOUR CIRCADIAN RHYTHMS

Why do circadian rhythms matter? They explain why the best times to study are in the morning when the prefrontal cortex is activated, as shown in this diagram.

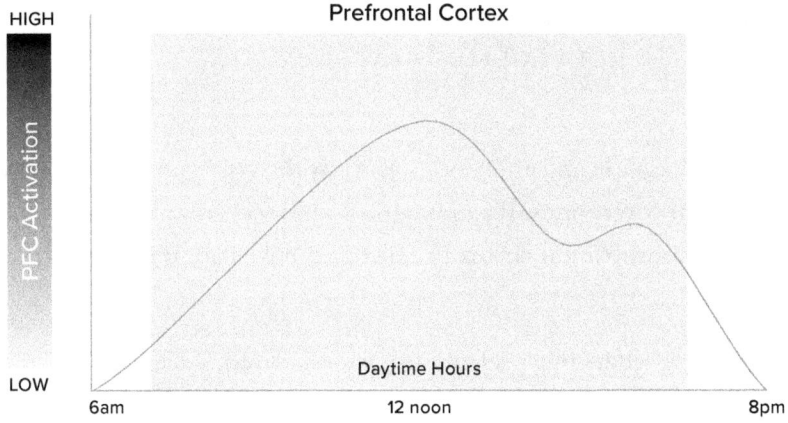

TIME TO MEET YOUR PREFRONTAL CORTEX

The prefrontal cortex is the source of problem-solving and decision-making. It activates from the time you wake up in the morning to a peak at about midday. Then this activity starts to taper off. There's usually a dip sometime between 2 and 4 pm. Some nations, such as Mexico and Spain, have a siesta time in the afternoon because they know that the body is feeling sleepy. We all feel a little bit sluggish in the afternoon, especially after a big lunch. The prefrontal cortex activity elevates again slightly about 5 pm, and then gradually tapers down to the time when you go to sleep.

Teenagers are an exception to this rule. Until you are 20 or so, your circadian rhythm runs a couple of hours behind. I've heard educators say that high school shouldn't start before 10 am because teenagers' brains start activating from about 10 am onwards. However, if you are a medical registrar studying for exams, you will indeed be older than 20.

The idea of morning study is to take advantage of the prefrontal cortex activity to get more study done in a shorter period. This is what happens: you learn more in less time.

> The trainees I work with often report that morning study is at least equivalent to six or seven hours of study over the day.

Then, take a break in the afternoon (on your days off), and spend some time with your loved ones. It's not a good time to study. And you don't need an active prefrontal cortex to relax and have fun. It's better if you don't, in fact.

In the evening when the prefrontal cortex is tired, I suggest you test yourself. It might sound strange to examine yourself when you are tired.

I have found that this is when all the sabotaging thoughts come in: "I'm too tired, I can't do this." However, if you put on a timer and you know that you're going to evaluate yourself, you can usually do it. And this pressure is what it feels like when you do exams. Practise examining yourself at a time when you don't want to do it, and you've got all these negative, anxious thoughts in your mind. You will soon learn to be able to sit exams under pressure. Testing at night is the equivalent of exam pressure. Ask yourself this:

Do you want to be comfortable or do you want to be ready?

A surgical registrar described his relentless study routine. "What I used to do was get up about eight o'clock in the morning, have breakfast, do a little study from 10 o'clock to 12, take a lunch break, do another two hours from two to four. Then take another little break for half an hour or so, then I'd do another two or three hours." He was studying six to eight hours a day on his days off.

When he started doing just four hours in the morning, from 8 am to noon, he said, "I did what you asked me to do, and subjectively marked how effective my focus was over each hour. I noticed that when I did four hours in the morning, I got so much more done than when I did six or seven hours. I was able to focus during that time more readily." However, he usually had only one day off per week, or he might be on call every second weekend. Four hours of study in the morning on his one day off was not enough. He had to squeeze a little extra study in when he could, even on work days. Since he now knew that his brain worked better in the morning, he was quite selective about choosing when he would study.

NOW YOU CAN GET A GOOD NIGHT'S SLEEP

So, you have done your study, given yourself time to recover, and have done an hour of testing. How do you think you are going to sleep? I guarantee that you will feel happier, more relaxed and ready for a good night's sleep. When you use this system good quality sleep will enable you to learn well.

If you want to get up in the morning on your day off and study until noon, you need a good night's sleep, otherwise you will be too tired to concentrate. We don't fully understand why we need to sleep, even with the most recent research on the brain. We do know, however, that when we sleep, we set in stone material that we've learnt. We need to rest well to have quality learning that goes into long-term memory.

WHAT IS SLEEP HYGIENE?

Our bodies need a routine to get to sleep. There are several ways to signal to the body that it is time to wind down. When you get into a habit of study, rest, testing and sleep, you start to build what the experts call

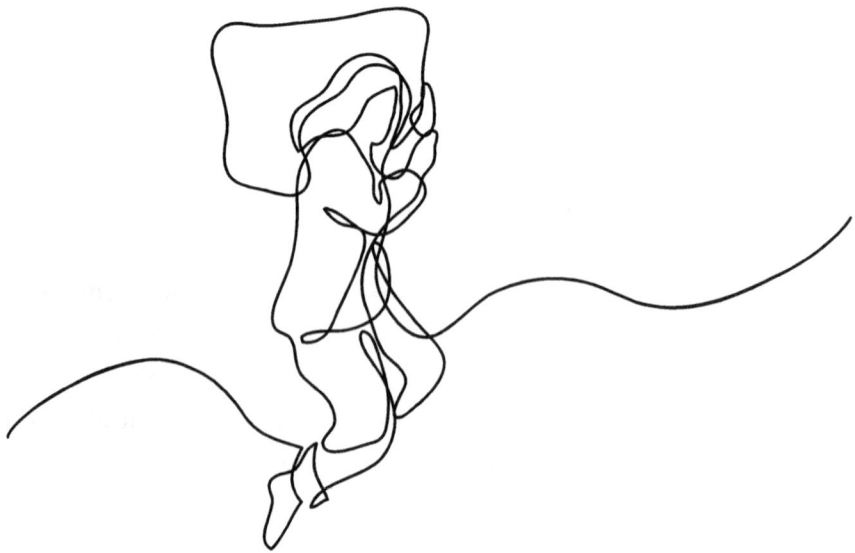

sleep hygiene. Everything we've learned about sleep has emphasised how crucial it is to our mental and physical health. Yet most of us probably sleep less than seven hours a night. This is less than it used to be before the proliferation of electric lights at night in the latter half of the 20th century, then the use of televisions, computers and smartphones in more recent years. It's certainly very hard to have good sleep hygiene when you do shift work with irregular hours.

It helps to turn off all your devices about an hour and a half before bed. That blue light on your screen robs you of the sleep-inducing melatonin. Darken your bedroom and maybe have a milk drink in the evening. There is tryptophan in milk that relaxes your body. Do your testing early in the evening. Don't test right up until the time you sleep. Increase your core temperature. Studies done at the Australian Institute of Sport indicate if you have a hot bath, which increases your core temperature, then rinse off with a lukewarm shower, the muscles relax, and you sleep better. Also, if you wanted to sleep better during the day after a night shift, then sit in bright sunlight for a few minutes before retiring to sleep in a darkened bedroom.

NUTRITION AND EXERCISE

It's surprising how many doctors I meet who do not eat well or do enough activity, especially when they are studying. I've already mentioned the surgical trainee who didn't eat for 24 hours. On a regular basis, she only had evening meals. She did not take breaks during the day. She didn't have breakfast at all.

Of course, doctors already know that the brain and the body need proper nourishment. You trained in this. The brain is not separate from the body; both need plenty of protein, a balanced diet, and exercise. Walking up and down stairs, and along the hospital's corridors is not enough. No, it's not!

Doctors tell me how fatigued they are. You have a right to believe you are tired because of all the work demanded of you. If you want to feel less fatigued, though, you've got to do a little extra. You've got to look after your body and brain.

Regular food is important. It is quite easy to have an orange or a banana or a handful of nuts on the run. Keep off sugar as much as possible because it leads to brain fog when you try to study, and too much sugar late in the evening is likely to keep you awake.

You don't need to set aside a significant slab of time to fit in exercise. Use your muscles in short bursts. You could just run on the spot or do push-ups.

Doctors are no exception to the rules on nourishment, exercise and quality sleep. We all need enough sleep to have the energy to exercise, and we need enough nutrition to have the energy to exercise. You can't ignore these things just because you're a doctor.

NO-ONE KNOWS BETTER THAN YOU

The consultants you work with might say you don't need to worry about all this. Just get down and study, find time for it. This is not helpful. Consultants forget just how hard it is to prioritise looking after yourself when you are a trainee. It might be 10 or 20 years since they were trainees. They've forgotten how gruelling the process is.

They might even say, "Just put all that self-care stuff on hold. Make study your priority." They will tell you that you need more than just your days off to do your study. You should study every evening and every day. I have seen again and again that this doesn't work. We know it doesn't work because of the failure rates in exams..

Because the quality of study in the evenings is poor, it can be mindless study. My clients who evaluate the effect of studying in the evening invariably point out that it is poor. They tell me that they can't remember what they reviewed the night before. A structure of study in the mornings on your days off only and testing yourself seven days a week on your exam components, usually after work, provides a bit of balance.

> You study when the brain is fresh, you test yourself under pressure when the brain is stressed.

And you make sleep, food, exercise, and family and friends a priority. You spend the afternoons of your day off on recovery.

HOW TO MEASURE YOUR RECOVERY

You will start to notice a difference straight away.

If you've got a weekend off, and you get your study done in the morning and then take the afternoon off, you say, "Wow! Gee! That felt good. I had some time off. I went out into the sun, I saw my kids, and I still did some study." If you do that on your days off every time, after about three weeks, it does become a habit.

I've had doctors who come back to me at the second visit and say. "This has made such a difference. I feel I now have a plan and I've got a bit of life back."

After about a week, start to test yourself on material you read earlier on your days off, and then evaluate your test. You will begin to see a difference. Around the hospital, people will say, "You look a bit happier," or, "You're talking a bit louder, and you're much clearer in your answers to my questions."

I remember how excited one doctor was when she first changed her study and testing schedule. She had told me that she really liked studying and had not had trouble passing exams. However, the main reason she had contacted me was that she wanted to give herself every chance of passing her final exam the first time, as she had a young baby. She did not want to fail and feel that her life with her partner and baby was on hold. I loved the email she sent to me after the first session we had together. This is an excerpt from it:

> It's amazing how re-framing the exam to 'a challenge' makes it much more enjoyable for me to study. I am going to follow your advice to the letter, so I can report back to you at the end of the week. My first 4-hour morning study period yesterday was an eye-opener… I was surprised at how much I can achieve in 50 minutes when I'm focusing [effectiveness of focus score] at around 8 or 9 out of 10. I've never taken 10-minute study breaks before. I usually keep going or go through for a few hours while I'm 'in the flow' until I find my attention wandering and then I take a break. So, I was dubious initially (and I felt a lot of internal resistance leaving the desk at 50 minutes, because I was focusing so well). But you're right! The regular breaks meant that I didn't hit the wall at three to four hours, and the last hour was just as productive as the first.

This doctor was delighted to be able to spend more time on her days off with her baby. Previously she would study most of the day and just take breaks for an hour or so to play with the baby. She continued to see me until she had completed her written and viva exams. She kept me on my toes, and I enjoyed working with her as she was so enthusiastic about what she was doing.

As mentioned before, there are three basic principles in my study system. The first principle is to learn about yourself, your needs, and how to recover, which is what we have covered until now. Later I will show you how to remember and understand the material, and how to attend appropriately and get your message out there in written and oral form. Also learning the art of engaging others.

But first recovery. Unless you get a better life-work balance, then the brain isn't going to work optimally. My system works because, as brain research indicates, the best learners are aware of how to study thoroughly, and then have the motivation and the strength, the mental strength, to make these changes.

Before you read further, let's see how stressed you are right now.

ARE YOU FEELING REALLY STRESSED?

Rate how you're feeling on the following scale:

	NOT REALLY	SOMETIMES	MORE AND MORE	MOST OF THE TIME
Increased fatigue	1	2	3	4
Increased irritability	1	2	3	4
Loss of enthusiasm	1	2	3	4
Feel less competent	1	2	3	4
Tense and tired most of the time	1	2	3	4
Decreased tolerance levels	1	2	3	4
Can't fall sleep or disturbed sleep	1	2	3	4
Lower self-confidence	1	2	3	4
Overwhelmed by "stuff"	1	2	3	4
Not enjoying life	1	2	3	4

(Adapted from Thayer, R. E., 1986)

If you scored between 30 and 40 points, then you need to act.

ACTION PLAN

✓ Have these useful study tools on hand: recording device, diary, digital timer, headphones, interval timer.

✓ Study for four hours before noon on days off (see Chapter 4 for details).

✓ Test specific exam components of your choice daily after work (See Chapter 5 for details).

✓ Ensure you have good sleep hygiene, good nutrition and regular exercise.

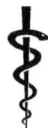

CHAPTER FOUR

ATTENTION LEADS TO BETTER STUDY

"Success is nothing more than a few simple disciplines, practised every day."

JIM ROHN

In this chapter, I explain the two parts of your brain that must work together for you to pay attention well. Then we will look at how you can motivate yourself to stay focused. I'll give you some tips for maintaining concentration right up to your exam. Focusing your attention on what is relevant is the key to success in exams. Focused attention enables you to integrate, synthesise and set material into long-term memory.

Since you are going to spend less time studying, you must make sure it's good-quality study. Why waste time on poor-quality learning, ignoring family and other social needs? Make your study time valuable, and then you can spend less time studying, and more time enjoying life. If you don't – and I have seen this – you will become burnt-out. You'll be exhausted and unmotivated.

If you focus your attention, you will commit facts to long-term memory more effectively because you are using the right techniques. You learn the material when you are fresh. You are not trying to cram details in at the last minute before the exams.

The key to success is "deliberate practice". Deliberate practice refers to practice that is purposeful and systematic. It requires focused attention and is conducted with the specific goal of improving performance. Deliberate practice takes advantage of the brain's ability to respond when pushed to its limits. If you have already had a day at work, you have had up to 15 hours on your feet. You are pushed to the limits; you are fatigued. If you test under conditions like that, you put yourself under pressure. It is not pleasant, but that deliberate practice makes all the difference. You want to achieve more control over every aspect of your performance.

Deliberate practice has two main components:

- paying attention to what you are doing
- concentrating on those aspects of your performance that you find most difficult.

It doesn't matter what kind of performer you are – a musician, an athlete, a doctor, a university student – deliberate practice is the most important and potent way to prepare for any performance. For example, to achieve higher levels of control over every aspect of performance, an elite diver breaks up what looks like a continual performance into little pieces, perhaps focusing on the approach and hurdle when on the springboard or spending time on entries into the water; maybe working on a specific dive that is not yet consistent, or perhaps spending time on their least favourite dive.

The key is to practise things that are not yet working well, so that the overall performance is improved.

Be prepared to toss out strategies you have used in the past. Especially if they haven't worked for you. But that's sometimes quite hard. If you used to study from 9 am to 6 pm, that can be frightening to toss out. You might feel that and studying only four hours is not enough. But I can assure you it is enough. It works because you work with your brain, and not against it.

HOW THE PREFRONTAL CORTEX AND THE AMYGDALA WORK TOGETHER

Understanding how the prefrontal cortex and the amygdala work together to focus and direct attention is essential if you want to apply the structured study approach in this book. Getting these two parts of the brain working together is the first step to getting your attention focused on your study.

The amygdala is an ancient part of the brain that responds quickly to threats. Even before you consciously perceive a threat, your body is primed for fight and flight by the amygdala. Your senses heighten. The amygdala doesn't wait for you to respond consciously. That is something humans have always needed, in an evolutionary sense, and we still need. If you step out onto a road and then see a car coming, the amygdala lets you respond quickly, without thought. It is a shortcut that allows the body to react in an emergency. It's useful at times, but it needs to be controlled. It's not much fun always being stressed.

When you become aware of a threat, and this is at least half a second after the amygdala fires up, your prefrontal cortex can then tell the amygdala to quieten down. The prefrontal cortex controls the amygdala. I like to use the analogy of the amygdala being like a nervous horse that gets spooked easily, and the prefrontal cortex being like an expert rider. When the horse rears up, the rider has strategies to calm the horse and get it under control. If you've learnt some techniques to calm yourself, and if you've been practising them in a safe environment, then you can control the factors that cause your amygdala to fire up.

An example of the amygdala and prefrontal cortex working together is when you see or do something you fear and yet the outcome is safe. Your prefrontal cortex will store the memory, and you can use the memory of safety to calm the amygdala in future. There are other techniques, such as diaphragmatic breathing, that will soothe the amygdala and the fear response. If you store enough safe memories through repeated deliberate practice of material you don't like, then you can control your anxiety.

You might be wondering how anxiety relates to attention? It is preferable to have an optimal level of body activation for each task we complete. Think of optimal body activation as homeostasis, where our body and brain are working well together, and then when body activation increases above an optimal level our body goes into survival mode where we tend to experience negative or distressing emotions and feelings. The higher your body activation above an optimal level for the task, the more likely you are to feel a negative emotion such as anxiety, and the lower your attentional capacity to the task.

For example, an elite pistol shooter needs a low level of body activation so that her hand doesn't shake and she can aim accurately at a target. However, a defensive player in rugby would benefit from higher body activation to tackle members of the opposing team. Just think about an example closer to home. I'm sure there are times when you get angry with a family member or close friend. When you become highly emotional, you find that you can't conduct a logical argument as well as you can if you keep calm. It's much the same with performance anxiety over exams. It's harder to access the material you know when asked questions.

Think about that jittery horse. When it gets a fright, it runs in any old direction. It's not paying attention to where it's going. It's up to the rider to bring the horse's focus back and say, "We're going in this direction". The more you practise strategies that calm down that horse, the better the attention to a task.

PRACTICAL WAYS TO INCREASE FOCUS AND ATTENTION

REMEMBER WHY YOU ARE PUTTING YOURSELF THROUGH ALL THIS STUDY

Every student needs to have a strong "why" – a reason that drives them to do their exams. If you want to succeed, your why needs to be stronger than your why not. What don't you like about your life right now? What are you trying to change?

You need to keep this as a reference point. And then you can see and measure your progress away from what you don't like and towards what you want.

Sometimes you need to remind yourself why you wanted to become a doctor. Remember your passion years ago when you were allocated to work a term in a specific area of medicine? Do you remember how enthusiastic you were to learn as much as you could? You probably made a decision back then that this was going to be your chosen specialty, and your focus from then on was around research, clinical work, and teaching in that area. Your reality, once accepted onto the training scheme for that specialty, was that life became very busy and stressful. You weren't spending enough time with family and friends, and study and long work hours took over. This could easily become overwhelming, but it's important to keep your eye on the end goal – becoming a consultant with a career in your chosen specialty. You need to be realistic, focus on your weaknesses and strengths, and set aside a little time each day to learn more in preparation for those final exams.

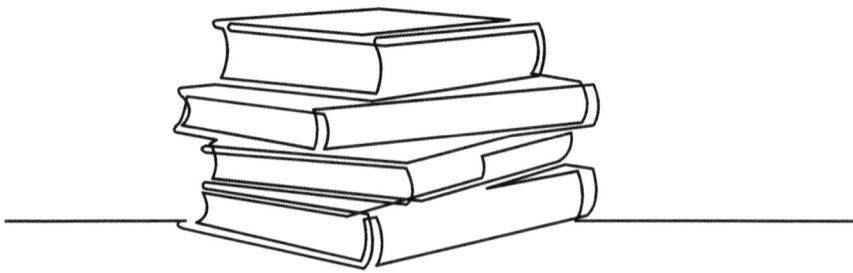

The closer you get to the exam, the stronger your natural motivation to pass becomes. In the early days, you will have to rely more on your why: the reason you want to change your life by doing these exams.

START SLOW AND GRADUALLY INCREASE YOUR STUDY LOAD OVER TIME

In the previous chapter, I talked about studying when the prefrontal cortex is most active, between 8 am and noon. That takes into account normal daily circadian rhythms.

Let's talk about the build-up towards your exams. If you are smart, you start studying several months before your exams. It is hard to maintain an intense study routine for months at a time.

Start slowly with your study and testing regime and expect it to be a bit hard at first. Changing from one habit to another habit is not easy. When you first make changes, you might relapse into your old habits. You might have a day when you think, "No, I can't do this." If you persist, after a month or so the new schedule becomes a habit and becomes much easier. As the Greek philosopher, Aristotle said, "Excellence is a habit; it is not an act."

Research shows that deliberate (structured and purposeful) practice is essential to managing stressful situations. You need to learn to deal with your negative thoughts about fatigue, feeling incompetent, failing. Under exam pressure, those thoughts become more prominent.

If you start in a more measured way in your study and testing regime, you won't experience too much failure or relapse. You'll keep positive about what you're doing. It is much easier to increase what you're doing when it's working, and you feel successful.

As you get closer to an exam, reduce the amount of studying and increase the amount of testing. In other words, increase the amount of deliberate practice of the components you will find in the exam. This primes the brain for the impending exam. In Chapter 6, I will give you detailed instructions for testing. For now, what you need to remember is to start slowly and build the intensity of your study and testing. As you get closer to your exam, shift the balance towards more testing.

For example, replace some of your morning study time by testing yourself on a topic you have previously studied. By the way, if you've had a crummy night's sleep or you've been out late, and you're sluggish at 8 in the morning, a short testing session under timed conditions will wake you up quicker than study.

Essentially, the aim is to create an exam condition as a non-unique situation.

This allows you to put more focus on responding with an appropriate answer rather than focusing on the exam structure. Examples of exam structure include the amount of time available, whether it is a "compare or contrast" question or a "discuss" or "list" question. With deliberate practice prior to the exam you will learn to recognise the type of question asked and will have developed a template for the type of answer required. Also, with practice, you will be comfortable in completing the answer within the time available for each question. Therefore, you can place more attentional resources on the responses to the questions rather than on the structure of the exam.

STUDY IN 50-MINUTE SPRINTS

Get out your digital timer. You'll need it to space out your study sessions. Set it to go off after 50 minutes and start your study session. When the alarm goes off, reset the timer for a 10-minute break. Then complete another 50-minute study session. Try and do four of these 50-minute study sessions, separated by 10-minute breaks, on your days off. Why do you need a timer? Because we all get on a roll sometimes, and we think we are working well. I have worked with doctors who swear they are studying efficiently when they sit at the desk for hours at a time. But what happens without realising it? Your attention to your study degrades over time. You end up doing less for a more extended period. You don't notice that your attention span has deteriorated until it's too late. It's important to keep the prefrontal cortex fresh. Your mind gets distracted and your attention wanders if you stay on the same topic for too long, and you don't take short breaks.

After 50 minutes on the first topic, leave the desk. Go to the toilet and get a coffee or tea. Do 10 push-ups or sit-ups. Anything. Put the clothes out on the line. Why is it necessary for you to leave your desk? That refreshes the attention of the prefrontal cortex. If you sit at your desk, what are you going to do? Look at your email? You are still doing screen time. No, take 10 minutes to do something more active, and you will be fresher and more able to study. If you need to, this is the time to check your phone or answer a phone call. A text might have come in that you're dying to answer. Go for it.

But after 10 minutes, when your little timer goes again, you're back at your desk, ready, fresh for the next topic.

CHANGE TOPICS HOURLY

It's essential to change topics hourly. That's right. Keep in mind, you want to keep the prefrontal cortex fresh, and your attention at the maximum level while you study. If you spend four hours on one topic, your prefrontal cortex starts to disengage.

Get your topics organised the night before. Don't fluff around at 8 am; work it out the night before. Otherwise, you waste half an hour in the morning. Plan the four topics you intend to cover, then spend your first 50-minute sprint on one topic, take a 10-minute break, and then switch to another topic.

START WITH THE TOPICS YOU DISLIKE

After you have set out the topics you intend to study, rank them according to which ones you like the most. Then start your study sprint with the one you dislike the most! How often do we avoid doing what we dislike? We immediately go to a topic we like, and we don't get to the topics we dislike. So always start out with a topic that's not your favourite and move towards the topics you enjoy. This will keep the prefrontal cortex a bit more focused.

RATE HOW EFFECTIVELY YOU STUDY

In your paper diary (that I advised you to buy in the last chapter), monitor the effectiveness of your attention to your study. It will help with your motivation. Research indicates that monitoring progress – how you're going – is motivating.

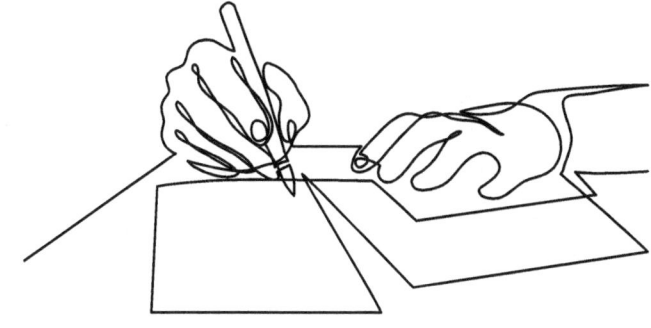

Swimmers sometimes have a whiteboard at the end of the pool. Every time they do a 200-metre time trial, for instance, they get out and put their time on the whiteboard. Then they get back in and do it again. Logging their own time on the whiteboard has been shown to increase their chances of improving.

Self-monitoring allows you to assess your behaviour to determine the competence of your response. It also provides a benchmark by which to compare any subsequent action. That becomes self-reinforcing, as you recognise behaviour change, which motivates further change.

At the end of your 50-minute study sprint, rate how well you attended to the topic during the period. Write a score in your diary with one being poor, and up to 10 being excellent. Don't rate how much work you did, just how well you were able to focus. Were you looking at two flies climbing up a wall, or were you wondering what to cook for dinner? Or were you focusing on the subject? If you score six or above, then your focus on the topic is adequate. If you score five or less, it may just be a one-off. However, if a pattern emerges and you are always distracted from study at a specific time of day, this may need to be examined more closely.

As soon as you implement this program, you will see those attentional focus scores start to track up. You will begin to feel far more in control of what you're doing.

TWO SUCCESS STORIES

I found one dermatology registrar to be extremely conscientious. She did nearly everything I suggested. She loved doing the work, was very enthusiastic, but she found it hard to stop when she was on a roll. There was a bit of resistance there. She just felt, "Oh, I'm doing so well, I'll keep going!" She either wasn't taking a 10-minute break, or she'd maybe take five minutes off after she'd been working for an hour and a half. I noticed she was giving herself only one score for attentional focus for the four hours of work in the morning. Because she did not break it down to four scores, this registrar was not aware that her attention may have been diminishing over the time. I persuaded her to rate her attention hourly, and then to stick to the breaks. She had to admit, a few weeks down the track, that it made a difference to the quality of her attention over the four hours.

An intensive care registrar came to me at his second session saying, "This isn't working for me." I was baffled, so I asked him more questions to see what he was doing. Here's what I found out: he was tweaking the sessions. He was studying right up till 1.30 pm. He wouldn't start till 9 am. He had longer rest breaks. He'd be out for 15 or 20 minutes. He took time out for a late brekkie, which is okay if you schedule it in. I also found out he wasn't monitoring his sessions. He just had a general feeling, "Oh, this isn't working for me." But, in fact, he wasn't sticking to the schedule in any way.

By the time he came to the third session, this registrar had really tried to make it work, and he had changed his mind. He'd stuck to the schedule and watched his attention scores climb.

RECORD YOURSELF AND PLAY IT BACK

In the next chapter I explain in detail that any reading you do in your study sessions should be active not passive. This involves recording the responses to five or six questions for each hour of study that you complete. Everybody dislikes listening to the sound of their voice (well nearly everybody), including me. But this is one little piece of technology you must use, no matter how painful it is. When you record your voice on your smart phone, and monitor progress in your paper diary, you will get feedback that nobody else will give you. Consultants are too busy listening to the content to focus on how you're responding.

It's easy to record. The doctors I work with do it well. They are conscientious about recording. What they don't do, later, is listen to themselves. And they will bring up every excuse under the sun not to listen to the recording.

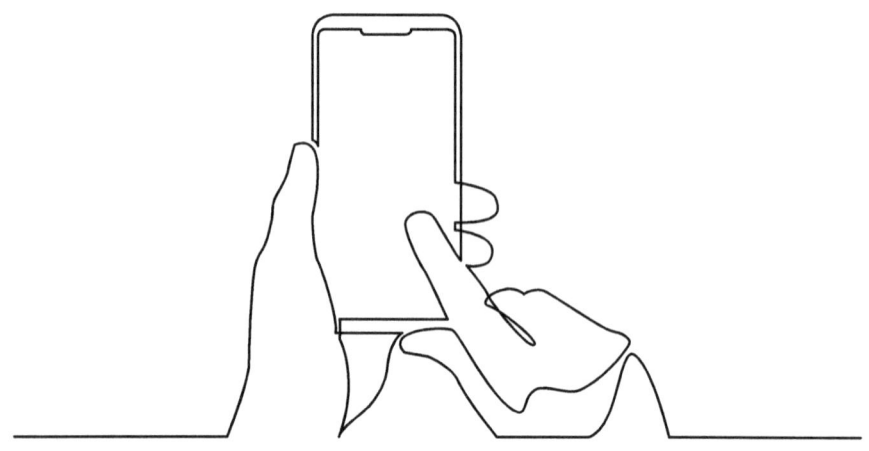

But only by listening to the recording, will you understand.

You will see, "Oh, I used 100 words then, instead of 10. I was not succinct. I was not clear. I prevaricated. I did not get my message across." This way, you learn these things by listening to yourself, and you give yourself feedback. Then you won't get embarrassed by other people listening to you making this kind of mistake in your exams, or in your discussions with consultants.

If you have a partner or friend who is keen to help, an extra pair of ears to listen to your recorded test responses is invaluable. That partner or friend also feels that they are doing something constructive to help you prepare for your exams.

Self-evaluations may be entirely negative at first. I always tell registrars, "Look. You're not going to like the sound of your voice. But start at the bottom and work up. You will improve. Pretend you're a consultant listening to this voice." I sometimes ask my clients to record on their phone a response to a question from me. When they listen back to the recording, they are quite astounded at how poorly they responded.

USE ALL YOUR SENSES TO HELP PAY ATTENTION

There is a science behind how the brain learns optimally. And brain research indicates when we involve all our senses in learning – sight, sound, smell, touch and taste – we commit more material to memory. We need to pay attention to our senses. Too often they are outside our awareness. There is a quote from *The Motorcycle Diaries of Che Guevara*, that says, "If you can see, look. If you can look, observe." That is really paying attention. How often have you been introduced to someone, and a few moments later you can't remember their name? It's an example of where we are not paying attention to our sensory input.

For instance, in the United States, a seven-year-old child might have a vocabulary of about 6,000 words. If they go into a national spelling bee competition, that same child might develop their vocabulary to about 20,000 words. The way they do it is to use their senses and to attribute meaning to each word. They might use their sense of sight to spell out a word on a Scrabble board. Then they sound the words many times over. And then they give the word meaning. And, according to research by Beck et al. in 2002, by using those senses – sight, sound, and attributing meaning to the word (and of course attention increases with interest in the meaning of the word) – material is committed to memory.

So, reading an answer, listening to your voice giving that answer, and understanding the meaning behind the answer is increasing your chances of embedding that information into long-term memory.

ATTENTION IMPROVES WITHIN WEEKS

Clients tell me they are quite surprised at the fact that merely putting a timer on stops them from procrastinating. They don't suffer as many sabotaging thoughts. They see an improvement in their attention scores within a week.

Their partner comments, "Gee, you're sitting down at your desk more readily. You're even staying there!" Or a consultant might say, "Hmm. You sound a little bit better." You will feel a sense of increased wellbeing; you have control over your destiny. You won't feel quite as overwhelmed.

CRITICS

You might think my attention to detail is a bit obsessive. Plenty of people have told me so! For instance, I knew a junior doctor doing the anaesthetic Primary exam who thought it would be okay to cram for the last four weeks before his exam. He thought that would be enough to wing it and get through the exam. Now, to make it through academic life, most of us do what is called "massed practice", which is better known as cramming. We think, in the last few weeks, we're going to cram as much information into our heads as possible. However, that's not a way our brains like to absorb information.

And I had to remind this doctor that he might remember the information for the next couple of days, but in a week or two, the details would become fuzzy and even go completely. He was going to need to remember this information when he became a consultant. I pointed out to him that to learn the material properly would increase his performance and improve his career. It's not about cramming.

That means starting a good study practice four to six months out from the exam. Space it out. Bear with me, and you will find it works. Each step in my system leads to the next. Start with recovery, and then improve your ability to pay attention.

Of course, there are times when you have to be flexible with the system. Sometimes, you have no one to look after the kids, or you have to take them to school or day care. Perhaps clinical meetings are scheduled on your study day, or you are on-call for the weekend. Surgeons, in particular, work rigorous, long hours and have few days off. They need to study and test when they can, but at least reading this book makes them aware of the principles of good study practice.

Adapt the program when you must and then return to the routine as soon as you can. Be aware of the principles and use the prefrontal cortex when it is most activated. Increase testing closer to exams. The first step is to set an overall plan. Then, when a day comes up where you must take the kids to day care, and your partner can't do it for you, find another time when you can study.

For instance, an obstetrics and gynaecology registrar told me she was registered to be on-call on one of her days off for four weekends in a row coming up to an exam. She was about two or three months out from the exam. But she didn't start work until 8 am. I suggested to her, 'Why not go in at 7 am and do an hour's study in the morning, away from any distractions at home, before you start work?' That way, she got five hours of study, Monday to Friday, which at least made up for the day on the weekend when she could not study. She then worked out that there were other ways where she could adapt, be flexible, and still adhere to a useful study program.

SUMMARY

- Remind yourself regularly why you want to pass the exams ahead. What part of your life do you dislike and want to change? Keep this desire front and centre as you go through your study program.

- Understand that now you have set aside the mornings on your days off from 8 am to noon for study, you have given yourself a holistic life plan, in which study takes a specific place. This means you are no longer trying to do two things at once, like read to the kids and worry about studying in the same moment. No. You now do one thing at a time: study first, then rest, then test in the evening.

- Be precise about the hours and shift the tasks according to your proximity to the exam. The closer you get, the more you focus on testing. Use all the techniques to maintain attention. Work in 50-minute sessions, then break for 10 minutes. Change topics every hour. Start with the topics you dislike. Check your progress in your ability to concentrate by giving yourself a score between one to 10 in your diary.

- Learn a little bit how the brain works, and how to focus your attention. If you understand this, you increase your ability to understand the study material and embed this material into your long-term memory.

ACTION PLAN

✓ **Study in 50-minute sprints on days or mornings off work.**

✓ **Take 10 minutes break between study sprints.**

✓ **Change topics each 50 minutes, start with the least liked topic.**

✓ **Rate effectiveness of each study sprint out of 10.**

✓ **Record and listen to your responses (see Chapter 5 for details on active reading).**

✓ **Self-evaluate those responses –**
  a) for content
  b) for voice tone.

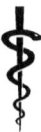

CHAPTER FIVE

HAVING YOUR BRAIN WORK FOR YOU AND NOT AGAINST YOU

"Overthinking can lead to self-sabotage and poor performance."

ANON

In this chapter I explain specific techniques, including pre-performance routines, active reading, mindfulness, energy regulation, thought stopping and using imagery, to perform at your best. It is important to carefully follow the steps given. You are changing the circuitry in your brain. Don't take any shortcuts. If you follow the instructions and practise conscientiously, then the techniques are more likely to work.

I have selected specific mental strategies described in this chapter because they build key areas essential in the training of doctors, and their individual needs. Mental skills training helps doctors develop mental toughness. Mental toughness is the use of a variety of mental skills which, when practised and used successfully, encourages unshakeable self-belief, resilience, motivation, focus, and the ability to perform under pressure. There is also an increased ability to manage emotional and physical pain.

The brain's ability to change in response to experience is the key to understanding the brain's development. This is called neural plasticity, and even though you're now an adult, you can still take an active part in influencing your brain's plasticity. In fact, the brain continues to evolve throughout life, and how it evolves depends on your experiences. If you understand this, you will be more motivated to approach learning in a scientific way. You will find it less frustrating. Your focus will be better, and you will waste less time trying out other approaches that don't always work. The techniques I recommend will improve your cognition, and help you avoid ruminating or having sabotaging thoughts. You will get a sense of calm and feel more in control. Before I go into this, let's look at whether you are suited to being part of a study group.

IS A STUDY GROUP RIGHT FOR YOU?

Some consultants recommend study groups. Many registrars have study groups and they can be very useful. Or they may waste valuable time. To judge if a study group is right for you, get a sheet of paper and draw a line down its full length. On one half list the advantages of being in a study group and on the other half list the disadvantages. When you look at these lists, do you feel you can justify being in a study group?

When overseas-trained consultants come to Australia, they need to sit the Australian Fellowship exam to practise here. I worked with one of these overseas-trained consultants. This poor guy had failed his Fellowship exam three times. He was in a study group on each occasion. At each of the exams most of the members of his study group passed while he continued to fail. He sadly remarked to me that previous members of his study group had now become his bosses. When questioned further he told me that he got a lot of satisfaction out of teaching the members of the study group what to do! He didn't focus on what he had to do to

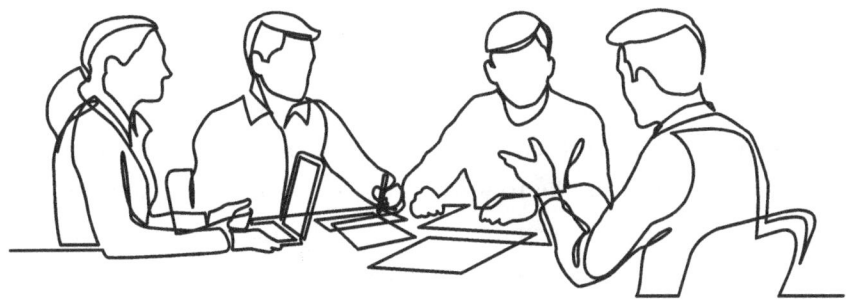

get through the exam. For him, it was not an advantage being in a study group. He put the teaching of others above his own needs.

A study group might be useful, or it might not. One factor depends on whether you are extroverted. Try answering this short questionnaire.

HOW OUTGOING ARE YOU?

1. **Assume something very embarrassing happened to you and it was noticed. How would you handle it? Would you:**
   a. treat it as a joke?
   b. blush or get angry?
   c. deny that it happened and fabricate some story?

2. **If you had some time off on the weekend would you prefer to:**
   a. be quite alone?
   b. share it with a close friend?
   c. be with some interesting acquaintances?

3. **Tonight is free – no study! Would you like to:**
   a. go to a party or popular night spot?
   b. watch some TV or read a book?
   c. have dinner with someone whose company you enjoy?

4. **Do you find yourself worrying about:**
   a. nothing very much?
   b. only things that are important to you?
   c. almost everything you think of?

Score: 1. a5, b3, c1   2. a1, b3, c5   3. a5, b1, c3   4. a5, b3, c1

If your score is:

16 or more: You have an outgoing personality and you like to have people around you. In fact, you tend to get bored or irritable when you are by yourself too long. You like to work in a study group, as it helps to give you structure with your personal study. You also like to bounce ideas off other people and it gives you confidence to see how you compare with the others.

9 or less: You like being on your own and can keep yourself occupied quite happily without the need for company. You probably have a good study routine, and dislike meetings where you present material to your colleagues. If others in the group don't pull their weight this is irritating.

10 to 15: You're right in the middle – not too extroverted and not too introverted. Being a member of a study group, and spending time on your own personal study are equally attractive to you. You like a good study group, but if the dynamics of the group are poor, you're fine on your own.

YOU ARE CHANGING THE CIRCUITRY IN YOUR BRAIN

When you have a lot riding on your performance, rely on science, not on hearsay. You wouldn't practise medicine based on hearsay, would you? You look for evidence. My techniques are evidence-based. With deliberate daily practice over at least three weeks, change becomes evident. Like any skill, you need to practise constantly before you get a result. Don't expect to have results in two or three days; it doesn't happen. What I've been told by many doctors, is that their hospital colleagues and/or their families, notice increased confidence or calmness under pressure even before they do. If you monitor these techniques and record scores in your diary, you will notice improvement over time.

Listen respectfully to what consultants suggest you should do regarding study, and then think about the methods suggested here. Be prepared to make some changes. You want to perform better. If you only partially follow the tips, the results will not be as good. Be prepared to follow instructions closely for any given technique to maximise the chances of it working for you.

PRE-PERFORMANCE ROUTINES

Pre-performance routines are rarely considered as a way of preparing for exams. Yet all elite athletes use pre-performance routines before they perform a difficult skill. And pilots would never let their planes lift off the ground without going through pre-performance routines.

Why do people use pre-performance routines when their performance is critical? As athletes would say, it's so they can "get in the zone", meaning they can focus their attention onto the skill they are about to perform. If you are facing a written exam, with components such as essays or short answer questions (SAQs), a simple pre-performance routine will help you focus your attention onto each word of the question. You will then be able to think clearly about the steps you need to take to select the best response. This routine can be used effectively before you respond to a written question. It can be modified for verbal responses.

A pre-performance routine is a very short activity you do before you respond to a question or before you do any task. For example, in soccer, when preparing to kick a penalty shot, perhaps a player will rub his or her hands, position their feet, consciously take a deep breath, and then kick the ball. That is their personal pre-performance routine. It enables the player to have full focus on endeavouring to successfully kick the ball into the net.

What goes on in our brains when we have a pre-performance routine? The brain responds positively to repetition. Because it is a repetitive routine and is something you've done thousands of times, you stay in your comfort zone. It's almost as though it is a security blanket.

The adrenalin doesn't increase above a level appropriate for the task, which would diminish your attentional capacity. This means you stay calm.

Imagine if an anaesthetic consultant nearly had a car accident on the freeway coming to work. Her adrenalin is high because she has had a major fright. Then she comes into the theatre and gets ready to mix drugs to make her patient unconscious for an operation. She is still shaky from the near miss on the freeway. Without a pre-performance routine, she could mix drugs incorrectly. In fact, the medical college to which anaesthetists belong has specific guidelines for mixing drugs, prior to operations, and it is expected that all their members will follow what is really a pre-performance routine.

Every college has different types of exams, both written and verbal. Written exams might include one-hour essays, half-hour essays, short answer questions of varying lengths, multiple-choice questions of various types, or extended matching questions. Some of these components may be on computer. Verbal exams also include different components. These may be cross-table vivas involving examiners or actors; or perhaps seeing real patients, obtaining histories and examining them, under various timed conditions, then later presenting to examiners. Perhaps the candidate sits in front of a computer to study images or look at x-rays while being questioned.

Your pre-performance routine will change depending on the exam component. Here are some examples:

- In a paper exam, take a deep diaphragmatic breath then underline the verb and the key words, and where relevant write sub-headings for the various points you want to make.
- In a computer exam, take the breath and write down the verb or any key words on a piece of paper.

- In an oral exam, take a deep breath before answering a question to allow yourself to collect your thoughts.

Not all exam components require a full pre-performance routine. Some components are too short, a full routine would waste time and energy. For example, most routines include a deep diaphragmatic breath, but with multiple-choice questions you wouldn't want to take, a deep diaphragmatic breath before every answer. You'd quite possibly hyperventilate. You would take a breath after every second or third answer just to maintain equilibrium, or, if perhaps you were a little unsure about your answer, you would take a breath and read the question again.

**By taking a breath,
you slow down and become calmer.**

Whatever your pre-performance routine, you must practise it every time you do an exam question. All the pre-performance routines I suggest include a diaphragmatic breath. The reason you take a deep breath is because it slows down your heart rate by five or six beats per minute. This brings your body back closer towards homeostasis, which is when your body is stable. Your adrenalin increases if you feel a bit overexcited or overanxious on a question. By taking a breath, you slow down and become calmer. Then you can attend more closely to your response, and you are more likely to draw the answer you want from your brain.

ACTIVE READING

Most people read passively, but "active reading" is the best way to learn facts. Active reading is deliberate practice that enhances your memory of the facts. Here is a breakdown of how it works:

- Have a pad of paper next to you in your study sessions.

- When you see a fact and think, "Oh, I need to remember that," turn the fact into a question and write it down. Then add the page number where you read the fact, so you can return to it later when you test yourself.

- In each 50-minute reading period of your four-hour study sessions, try to find five or six facts to turn into questions, that's about one page of questions per period. Let's say you had two days off, and each day you did four hours of study in the morning. That would be eight hours of study, resulting in eight pages of questions.

- Place these pages in a folder. Don't be tempted to answer the questions within 24 or 36 hours, as it is likely the answers would still be in working memory.

And here's how to test yourself five days later, after a work shift, when the answers are out of working memory.

- Take out the first page and record your answers to the questions on your phone.

- Open your text or study notes at the page number for the first question and read the fact as you play back your recorded answer. Then give a score for content from 1 to 10 for its accuracy. Mark all questions on the page for content.

- Then play back the answers again, and this time listen to the voice – does it engage you? Is it succinct and clear? If you answered correctly the voice is probably loud and confident. If you answered with some hesitation the voice probably mumbles, waffles, and sounds very unsure. Give yourself a score from 1 to 10 as to how the voice sounds. *Hint: Pretend it's not you you're listening to. Nobody likes the sound of their own voice.*

* Asterisk any answer with a low score, and revise at one of your study sessions.

If you have eight hours of reading a week, then do a sheet of questions each night. It should take about 15 minutes. If it takes longer, then your questions may be too complicated. You'll need to do two sheets on one of these nights; there are only seven days in the week!

There are four good reasons for doing this active reading and testing:

1. It's revision of reading from the previous week.
2. Multiple choice questions are just facts, and they are usually taken from the prescribed texts to avoid ambiguity.
3. All short answer questions are made up of facts, even if it's a clinical scenario.
4. This is good practice for the viva exams. You soon learn to make your voice sound confident and loud, once you hear how you sound when you're not sure about your answer.
5. You learn what you don't know, not what you already know.

Stick to the facts. When I ask my clients to choose a fact and turn it into a question of only one or two lines maximum, they often think "more is better" and they write a question that requires a long and involved answer! Then they come back to me and say, "I don't like this. It doesn't work. I recorded my answers, but it took me three-quarters of an hour to do five or six questions."

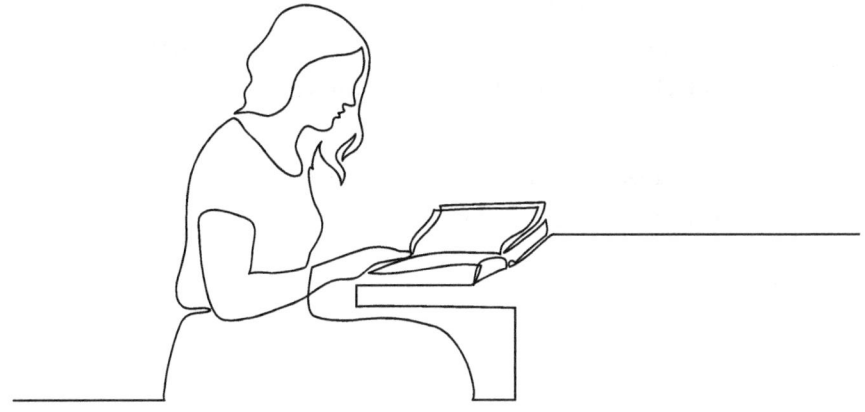

When I ask them, "How long is the question?" and they tell me, I fully understand why. What they've done is set themselves up for failure. They've made it too long. They're anxious, thinking about everything they need to remember. They forget that all they're doing is learning facts.

For example, perhaps you are reading about kidney function. There might be a long explanation and so you write a question like, "Describe the complete mechanism through which the kidneys filter the blood." That response would contain many facts. However, a fact within that explanation that you perhaps didn't know before could have been, "A secondary function of the kidneys is ..." This is one single fact, which you turn into. "What is a secondary function of the kidneys?"

Another example might be when reading about the drug Midazolam. Instead of writing a question such as "List all the requirements for using intravenous Midazolam," try something like, "What is the main requirement for the use of intravenous Midazolam?" The answer might be, "Every intravenous Midazolam administration requires resuscitation alert."

MINDFULNESS

Another area that is particularly important is staying in the present. How often during an exam or a study session, are you looking out the window, wondering how long before it's over, or thinking how little you know? You must have techniques to keep yourself in the present, so you are not worrying or thinking about your past and/or your future. You are staying where you ought to be.

Staying in the present keeps you calmer.

A growing body of research suggests that mindfulness, defined by Brown and Ryan (2003) as the propensity to be "attentive to and aware of what is taking place in the present", relates positively to one's ability to focus, maintain sustained attention, and can reduce anxiety during stressful events. These aspects have the potential to contribute to performance in medical exams.

Mindfulness is a technique to keep you focused on the present. Staying in the present keeps you calmer. Mindfulness is also a technique to use when you get overwhelmed with anything in life. It stops you ruminating about the past or the future. You stay in the present and enjoy the present.

I had a client, John, who had failed his exams on several occasions because, in his own words, he ruminated constantly. I thought I'd try a mindfulness technique with him. He liked it so much he went and discovered more about it, and decided he liked another technique even better. He then used that. His whole demeanour changed. He's calm. John now does a mindfulness exercise for about half an hour every day. His wife, a psychologist, has commented on his increased calmness under pressure.

Is that what I recommend? Not necessarily. Not everybody has a free half hour, but for him this was useful. It's something he enjoys, and it keeps him in the present. He continues to practise mindfulness even though he is now through his final exams and is a Fellow.

Another doctor told me a sad story about reading a book to one of his children at night. As he read, the child fidgeted. She was upset, and asked why he wasn't reading it properly? He was reading in a monotonous, boring voice, and I think she was aware that her daddy just wasn't "with her". The father realised he'd been thinking about his exam and his study, while he was reading. He wasn't in the present, he was not engaging his child in the story. It's important when you leave your study or work for the day that you spend quality time with your family or friends. Forget about your problems and focus on being in the present. Give yourself completely to whatever situation you are in. This doctor did try mindfulness and it made a difference. Even the fact that he realised he wasn't mentally "with" his child made him aware of how he managed his focus of attention.

There are some very good mindfulness apps around – from Headspace or Smiling Mind. However, because phones aren't allowed in the exam centre, these apps can't be used in the registration area, during a scheduled rest break, if you are quarantined, or when you are just waiting in the corridor. I use a "counting breath" to increase mindfulness under these circumstances.

COUNTING BREATH

This is where you breathe in through the nose to the count of three, and breathe out through the mouth to the count of six. For practice in the weeks or months leading up to the exam try and do at least eight to ten breaths at a time to allow the body and mind to relax. Do twice a day if possible and record its effectiveness in your diary. You will notice that the inhalation to a count of three and the exhalation to a count of six will encourage deeper breaths as you continue. You may also notice that the action of consciously counting will stop you from thinking of other things.

ENERGY REGULATION

Energy regulation is one of the most important techniques I teach. Energy regulation is your capacity to recognise your current energy levels and then control your energy when your body activates. As I mentioned in Chapter 4, the higher your body activation above an optimal level for a task, the more likely you are to feel a negative emotion such as anxiety, and the lower your ability to attend to the task.

Very often, people are stoic. They stifle their feelings and don't always recognise when they're anxious or angry until it's almost too late. They hold it in for as long as possible and then the emotion bubbles out almost uncontrollably. However, it is much better for your health and equanimity to have a technique to enable you to notice if your body is activating above a level that is optimal for a task, and then have a way to control that energy.

For example, you have two minutes to read a stem pinned to the door outside the examination room. This stem gives you crucial details relating to the patient inside. However, you find it difficult to concentrate your attention on these details. How do you know you feel this way? Well, the first indication is not in your brain; it's through activation in the chest. Your chest muscles tighten, and it feels as though there's a knot under the sternum. Perhaps this leads to tension out in your arms or hands, or up to the shoulders. Maybe you feel a drop of sweat trickle down your back. This is peripheral bodily tension and it distracts your thought processes. You start to feel anxious, as you still haven't been able to concentrate.

Another example might be just before you give a presentation to a group of doctors from different departments. You are nervous, and as you look around the sea of faces just before going up to the microphone, you forget what you had planned for your introductory remarks. You can't even remember the patient's name! You are tense, and your thoughts are racing, focusing mainly on how badly this presentation is going to be.

These would be two occasions when it would be ideal to use a centering breath: this is a deep diaphragmatic breath, but with a difference.

CENTERING BREATH

Practising a specific breathing technique, such as a centering breath, will help regulate energy by reducing the fight and flight response. Focusing on the breath lowers your heart rate so that you can concentrate more readily. It's one breath. It can be used whenever you become aware that your activation rate is too high, and you need to lower it.

There are three teaching points:

1. Feet flat on floor whether sitting or standing (the breath lowers the centre of gravity, which is why it's called a centering breath).
2. Breathe in and out through the mouth. You get more air into your lungs quickly as you inhale.
3. Total focus on the inhalation and exhalation of air from the lungs. By that I mean focusing on feeling the ribs expand and the lungs completely filling with air as you inhale, then the transition from inhalation to exhalation. Noticing that the shoulders relax; if sitting you settle deeper into the chair, and if standing you feel more grounded.

At the end of the exhalation there is a three-second window of opportunity, where there is nothing in the mind and one can direct attention to the task.

How do you know you have inhaled fully into the lungs? Place your longest fingers on each hand on top of your belly button. If your fingers come apart as you inhale, then you have breathed in properly, expanding your stomach muscles. It might help to watch in the mirror as you inhale.

To encourage automaticity of the centering breath, remind yourself every hour (by setting an interval timer), and at night record in your diary 2 scores from 1–10, for quantity and for quality of the breath.

TWO SUCCESS STORIES

An anaesthetic registrar told me about a difficult intubation where he successfully used this centering breath. As you probably know, an intubation is when you put a tube down the patient's throat to take over the breathing for the patient. Sometimes it is difficult if the patient is obese, or the throat opening is not as big as usual. This anaesthetic registrar had already tried once and failed. He was about to attempt the intubation again when, out of the corner of his eye, he saw his supervisor standing in the doorway, hand on hip.

Immediately his attention was divided. He thought to himself, "What the hell does she want? What's she watching me for?" His hands tightened up. His shoulders tightened up. He understood the risk was that he would not succeed the next time he tried the intubation. He stopped. For the next two seconds he took a deep diaphragmatic breath. He put his total focus of attention onto his inhalation and exhalation. At the end of the breath there was nothing in his mind. His hands were soft and pliable, and he was able to complete the intubation.

Then he attended to the supervisor. Was the supervisor judging the doctor? Probably not, it may have been a figment of his imagination. She just wanted to see him complete the intubation before talking to him. But his brain did not know if the threat was real or imagined. It activated just the same, causing his body to tighten up.

Last year, Stewart was sitting the oral section of the basic physician exam. He had apparently failed dismally on this exam component previously because of performance anxiety. I gave him the centering breath to increase his concentration onto his responses when questioned. At the second session, three weeks later, he said that this breath just wasn't working. He didn't have time to do it! I said to him "This is a breath. You have to breathe constantly, so how come you don't have time?" I had him go through everything closely, reiterating all the steps I had given him. He had not done them correctly.

Stewart had been asked to take a centering breath every hour for the 15 hours or so that he was awake. I had explained that the constant practice would mean that eventually he would automatically take a deep breath when he felt stressed. He'd not done the breath correctly, nor had he remembered to practise that breath hourly, which is quite likely if you don't have a way to remind yourself. He admitted he'd forgotten to get an interval timer to remind himself to take a breath. Consequently, he reported that he practised only five or six centering breaths daily. I had also suggested that Stewart use this breath around home – that it was useful to take a breath if he was irritated or frustrated by little things that family members did. He'd omitted to do that also.

After much persuasion, and with clear instructions from me just weeks out from the exam, Stewart began to practise the centering breath properly. He started to see results, especially when consultants commented on his improvement in practice vivas. He later reported, somewhat enthusiastically, that he had felt more confident, his performance anxiety was kept under control, and he'd passed the exam.

A centering breath is a brilliant technique to get back to the present. It focuses one's attention onto the task. And, of course, it can be part of your pre-performance routine as well.

THOUGHT STOPPING

As an exam gets closer, most people start having a cluster of persistent negative thoughts around the exam, particularly if they have failed previously. How often do you approach your exams thinking, "Oh gee, I'm going to fail again? What are the consequences?" If you have these persistent negative thoughts, you end up on a downward spiral and, in many instances, you don't even study. You think, "Oh, I can't do anything today, I feel so lousy. I'll wait until I feel a bit better." Then you feel guilty and down-hearted because you haven't done your study. This can spiral into general negativity; you don't feel like studying, that makes you feel even worse, and down you go.

A thought-stopping technique can reduce your negative thought patterns, especially when they're repetitive. It's important that you recognise the cluster of negative thoughts that form a pattern, and then practise this thought-stopping technique whenever the thoughts come to your consciousness. Here is a useful way to combat negative thoughts.

THE RUBBER BAND TECHNIQUE

Pick a repetitive thought or cluster of thoughts around a theme that comes up several times a day, such as "I'm going to fail again". Then think of a thought (or image or song) that inspires you and brings a smile to your face. It need not be related to anything to do with work or study. Once you have the two thoughts (one negative, and one inspiring and positive), get a rubber band and place it on your wrist. Whenever you think of failing, pull the rubber band out and ping it against your wrist (not too hard, but hard enough to sting a little). Immediately think of your inspiring thought. You will, with practice, begin to link your negative thought with the sting of a rubber band, and these thoughts will then lessen over time. Record in your diary how many negative thoughts you have daily and watch them diminish.

SUCCESS STORY

One doctor I worked with suffered from severe performance anxiety. She had some interviews coming up for jobs and had stuffed up her interviews on every previous occasion. She had a fantastic CV and her references were glowing. She always received an invitation to attend for an interview. However, interviewers just didn't want to employ her because she seemed so negative and unsure of herself. She was not herself at all when she presented at these interviews.

It was all related to her negative thoughts. She spent the whole interview thinking about how she was incompetent and no good. In the weeks before each interview, she'd be thinking to herself, "I'm incompetent, I can't do this, nobody wants me."

It seemed appropriate to give her a thought-stopping technique. I asked her to tell me about something that made her feel good. It took a little while, but you know what she said in the end? Singing Disney songs to her little girl. That made her happy. We didn't use a rubber band this time, as she was in theatre for much of the day. She couldn't wear one while operating. Instead, I asked her to gently bite the inside of her cheek or tongue whenever negative thoughts came to mind. Then she was to imagine singing Disney songs to her little girl.

When she first started doing this technique, she was thinking negative thoughts about 20 times a day. I asked her to record in a diary how many times she had to distract herself from the negative thoughts. The number of thoughts lessened in a little over two weeks. The key was she had to think of Disney songs to recalibrate her mood to one of positivity.

By the time she was invited to her next interview, she was able to have her negative thoughts under control. When she was sitting out in the waiting room ready to go in, she was more confident and relaxed; thinking of Disney songs had done the trick. She ended up getting one of the jobs she wanted.

IMAGINING SUCCESS

Imagery is using the senses to make your brain believe you are in the real situation itself. You can prove this to yourself right now. Imagine you have cut a lemon into quarters. You pick up one quarter of the lemon and put it in your mouth. You chew on the lemon. I bet that as you read these lines, and imagine chewing on the lemon, you start to salivate a little bit. The brain sends messages down to the salivary glands, which then excrete more saliva into the mouth to combat the stringent effect of the lemon juice.

The brain doesn't know the difference between you pretending to be chewing and you really chewing on a lemon. It's the same when you use imagery to improve performance. If you can imagine in detail doing something successfully, your brain doesn't know the difference.

If you imagine walking into a job interview confidently or performing a surgical procedure successfully – and if you do it often enough – the chances of real-life success are much greater. However, when using this technique, you must always practise in such a way that you imagine yourself performing to the best of your ability. If you can't do that each time you practise, then imagery is not for you. You must never ever imagine yourself performing poorly, as this will stick in your brain and you may then perform badly.

A typical example of an oral exam component to image might be a cross-table viva with two examiners present. Imagine walking confidently into the room, shoulders back, head up, and a relaxed expression on your face, instead of looking nervous and tense. Image the situation just before bed (when you are most relaxed, because this is when imagery is most vivid) using as many of your senses as possible to successfully handle the situation. Allow about 10 seconds to bring up the image, and then spend another 10 seconds or so practising walking confidently into the room and sitting down. Give a score from 1 to 10 for effectiveness of the image. Do the same imagery twice and record the best score in your diary.

Back when I was a performance psychologist for athletes, I worked with an elite gymnast. She came to me because she appeared to have lost the ability to do a specific skill in her trampoline routine. When she reached that part of her routine, she would blank out and her body would do something else. The manoeuvre she was trying to complete was called the "double in, half out". It's a forward double somersault with a half twist out to land on the feet. When she came to do this move, she wouldn't land on her feet. She'd land on her back. It was driving her crazy because she knew how to do it, but she had temporarily lost the ability to perform the skill.

I asked her to imagine doing the move. I asked her questions like, "What should your body do to land on the feet?" to get her to focus just on the technique she'd been taught. And she'd see it in her mind, "I kick my legs out straight".

I got her to imagine kicking her legs out and becoming aware of her heels, which is what her coach wanted her to do. She used kinaesthetic imagery: she felt in her body what she was doing. She imagined kicking the heels out successfully. Then, I asked her to imagine the skill that came before the double in, half out and add it on; then the skill after it. I asked her to image performing these three skills every night for about two weeks, and to give herself a score on how well she imaged it.

Many researchers have demonstrated that using the senses, and not just the visual, will enhance the use of imagery. I initially asked the athlete to practise this several times in our sessions with me present, to monitor that she was imaging correctly and was using senses such as touch, sight, sound, and kinaesthetic awareness, to increase the detail in the images. She became better at it. Soon she was again able to practise the skill successfully in her trampoline routine.

A word of caution on using imagery. It needs to be used wisely and carefully. Unless you are good at imagery, it's not something I would suggest.

Here's a way to tell if it is right for you. Close your eyes and imagine a piece of fruit, an apple. Now some people imagine that apple in full colour, others in black and white, and some see only the Apple logo. I suggest you only use imagery if you can see an apple in detail and in full colour. And always – this is something I must stress – always image positive situations because it's a powerful technique. You don't want to be imagining negative things happening.

HOW TO MEASURE THE SUCCESS OF THESE TECHNIQUES – CHOOSE THE RIGHT ONES FOR YOU

You don't need to use all the above techniques. Select what attracts you and suits your learning style and how far out from an exam you are. If you have only a month or so to go before your exam, select perhaps just one technique because there wouldn't be time to work on all of them. If you are a year out from the exam, you have time to experiment with different techniques and decide what you like and what works for you.

Researchers have found that monitoring progress in a diary increases motivation. This is why I suggest using your diary to monitor how often and how well you practise these techniques and score their effectiveness. You can score how many times you do them, what the quality is like, whether it is working.

Perhaps you might think to yourself, "Oh, goodness me. I have enough to do without practising all these techniques as well." But I would say, this. The techniques offered are all evidence-based. Research shows practising these techniques daily will increase focus of attention to the task. This increased focus will lead to enhanced performance over time. The techniques I have selected are ones that I find work well for my medical clients. With practice they will work for you too, and you will feel more in control.

ACTION PLAN

✓ Always use a pre-performance routine with essays and SAQs.

✓ Practise recording/listening daily to active reading questions from previous study sessions.

✓ Regularly practise mindfulness technique – use an app or the counting breath technique.

✓ Do the centering breath every waking hour to regulate energy.

✓ Reduce negative thoughts with the rubber band technique.

✓ Image successful medical situations – if you are a visually oriented person.

✓ Monitor effectiveness of each of the techniques on a regular basis

_____ mark from 1 to 10.

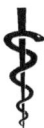

CHAPTER SIX

TESTING – PRACTISE UNDER PRESSURE TO PERFORM ON DEMAND

"Tell me and I forget, teach me and I may remember, involve me and I learn."

BENJAMIN FRANKLIN

In this chapter we talk about testing under speed-versus-accuracy conditions, the use of deliberate practice, which is purposeful and systematic, and the evaluation of your testing. All exam components in the medical exams need facts in the responses. You will learn strategies to revise, test, and evaluate those facts daily to keep them in the forefront of your memory. When you practise your exam components under pressure, you maintain control while you prepare for a major exam. Unless you practise under pressure, you will not experience what you may encounter in your exam. This system is designed to make practice a better simulation of your exams.

For instance, let's say you have 10 short-answer questions, each 10 minutes long, but you take 15 minutes to answer them because you want to write a good response. You will not learn what you need to learn – which is how to answer the question in 10 minutes – unless you practise under pressure. Practising under pressure could be always writing the responses in nine minutes, not 10 minutes.

This technique comes from my background as an athlete a long time ago. I was an elite springboard and high board diver. The closer I came to a competition, the more my coach made my practice like a competition. For example, a long way out from the competition, I did four or five of the same dives per practice, learning to make them better. Closer to the competition, I did one or two dives only. I did not have the luxury of trying to perfect my dives through multiple attempts. The pressure was to do them well the first time.

If you can self-generate some pressure – and speed-versus-accuracy is one way to increase that pressure – then you simulate what may happen in an exam. After all, you don't do exams at times you want to do them. You do them whether you have a headache, whether you feel sick in the stomach, whether you have a cold.

> You must sit the exam however you feel.
> Thus, testing yourself under time pressure is useful.

Time is a limited resource. Testing concentrates your time. You will do fewer hours at your desk. An hour of testing every day makes your brain think faster.

Testing helps you chip away a little bit every day, seven days a week. It is good preparation for the exam. In this chapter, I'll give you techniques to test yourself under pressure. Initially you may not like them, but they will prepare you well for both oral and written exams. Let's take a look at them.

FIND OUT YOUR EXAM COMPONENTS

When I speak to a client in November who has an exam in February, the first question I ask them is to describe in detail their exam components. Their answers often surprise me.

"Oh, I think I've a few short answer questions and multiple choice."

I say, "Okay how many short answer questions?"

"Oh, I must look that up."

I don't think that's good enough. You need to know how and what you will be expected to do. Then you can develop strategies that test your ability to answer that exam component.

HERE'S WHAT YOU NEED TO FIND OUT, AND THIS IS JUST FOR THE WRITTEN EXAMS!

- How many of your exams are written and are paper-based?
- How many of your exams are computer-based?
- How long is each exam component and at what time of day?
- How many SAQs do you have?
- How much time is allocated for each SAQ?
- Are there several parts to your SAQs?
- Is each part of the SAQ variably marked?
- Are the allocated marks shown on the paper?
- Do you have any reading time?
- Will you be asked questions about photos or images, and will your answers need to be typed or can you write?

- How many multiple-choice questions (MCQs) will you have to answer?
- Are they true MCQs, or do they include true and false questions?
- Do you have extended matching questions?
- Are your MCQs negatively marked?

RESOURCES THAT WILL HELP YOU PREPARE
MULTIPLE-CHOICE QUESTION DATABASES

There are "black banks" of MCQs, which are made when doctors come out of the exams and try to remember all the questions. They write down the questions and the answers. You can use those MCQs but keep in mind that the answers may not always be correct. But there are some legitimate databases from overseas. They're not necessarily MCQs that will be used in Australia, but they're similar. You need to practise answering MCQs as you would in an exam, even if they are not always on the material you will be tested on.

COLLEGE-PROVIDED PRACTICE EXAM PAPERS

Most colleges will provide practice exam papers based on essay type questions or SAQs from previous exams over the last 10 years or more. They do not usually provide MCQs as these types of questions are difficult and time-consuming to create.

IMAGES OR PHOTOS

Sometimes the colleges will provide photos, x-rays, CT scans and other images, as certain exam components require the trainee to describe what they see and answer specific questions. Doctors tell me that they have no problem finding copies that they can use for testing. They often have plain images with no labels in their texts, and these often have associated questions that can be used for recording and listening to answers. There are even books of these images with questions and answers. All these can be used for testing purposes.

RECORD YOURSELF

Recording is much harder than writing an answer because there is less time to prepare your thoughts. You must ad-lib and organise your thoughts very quickly. As mentioned in the last chapter, you need to listen twice to the recording you make. First listen to the content: the quality of the information you provided. Then listen again just to your voice, so you can hear what goes wrong when you answer under pressure, and what sounds alright.

EVALUATE FOR CONTENT

People often record themselves quite happily, but they're reluctant to listen to the recording. Everybody dislikes the way their voice sounds, but you'll get over it. If you don't record and listen to yourself, if you don't get used to your voice, when you talk to an examiner you cannot focus your attention solely on your response. Your attention will drift. How intelligent am I sounding? Is that approval on the examiner's face? It is difficult to focus solely on your response if you're asking yourself questions. Your attention is divided, and the chances are that your response will deteriorate. If you record regularly, you get used to listening to yourself.

This technique is primarily for oral exams, but it's still good for a written exam because you are ad-libbing and thinking much faster than if you have the time for your thoughts to go from your brain down to your fingers and through the pen to the paper.

Because you are an active reader (see Chapter 5), you will have learnt to record and learn facts seven days a week. These facts can then be inserted into your SAQs, or other exam components where you are testing yourself by recording your responses.

A surgical trainee, Sergi, came to me very shocked and angry when he failed his exam for the first time. He didn't believe the exam feedback that he didn't answer the questions. He complained bitterly. However, he eventually began preparing for his second attempt, which included recording for the first time his responses to written questions. After listening to his answers, Sergi realised that he missed out crucial facts or misinterpreted the question quite often. He became aware that his full attention was not always on his answers. He changed his attitude, was less angry, and became quite a fan of recording and listening to his responses.

EVALUATE FOR VOICE TONE

After you listen to yourself and evaluate the content, sit back with a glass of wine or a cup of tea and listen again to the recording. At first, you'll probably think, "Oh yuck, I hate the sound of my voice. This is awful." Try to forget that it is you. Pretend to be the examiner and listen to this male or female voice, then ask yourself the following questions:

- How much do I like that voice?
- Is that voice clear?
- Is it focused on the answer?
- Does that voice engage me?
- Does that voice get the message across?

This gives you information that you might not otherwise get. (Not many people will tell you that you sound boring.) Give your voice a score. The more you listen, the more you will self-correct. We don't like to listen to anyone boring – even ourselves!

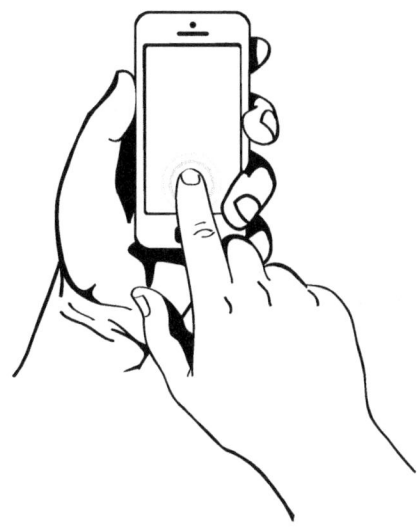

You may ask why it matters to be engaging and get the message across? If you have the facts, don't you pass? No, not always. Keep in mind that the examiners are evaluating trainees all day. They're human, they get tired. Your oral exam might be right before their lunch or at 4 pm, a terrible time of day. You need to learn how to speak and to engage your listener, because that encourages them to hear what you have to say.

Listening to the voice is one of the hardest techniques I get doctors to do. They will record, but they won't listen back to it. However, I make clients accountable for every piece of homework I give them. Once they start to listen objectively, they notice all sorts of quirks. They notice how they mumble. They notice they have a soft voice, or they squeak, or they answer in a monotone. You will start to notice these qualities of your voice, and once you are aware, you can change them.

RECORD AT WORK

If consultants ask you a question at work, record your answer on your phone. (You must ask the consultant's permission to record.) Then take it home and listen to it twice, once for content along with the consultant's feedback, and once for how you sound. If you find after listening to yourself that you are really dissatisfied, either with the content or the voice, then re-do your answer that evening while the material is still fresh. This will help cement in your brain the correct answer and how to get the message across.

Supanee, a physician trainee, spoke English with a strong accent. She always spoke too fast, and consequently the voice was monotone. It was hard to maintain focus while listening to her. When Supanee started listening to her recorded responses to consultants' questions, she was shocked. "I sound so boring – almost disinterested," she said.

Hearing her voice gave Supanee the impetus to slow down and pause at the end of her sentences when she recorded her future responses. She also started to concentrate more on "owning" the patient she was talking about. By "owning" the patient I mean pretending that she was responsible for the patient's welfare.

> Talking about the patient's care as though
> it is your patient, adds more colour and
> enthusiasm to your voice.

Consultants found it much easier to listen to Supanee and understand what she was saying. Now they did not overlook important points in her responses to questions.

EXAMS NEED FACTS

Exams need facts. You need to revise and test those facts daily to keep them in the forefront of memory.

Study always involves reading. Testing of facts always involves deliberate practice. Deliberate practice is the way to improve. This doesn't only apply to doctors; it applies to musicians, it applies to opera singers, it applies to athletes. You must have time to practise.

In the previous chapter, I talked about active reading. When you practise active reading, you turn the facts into questions. Then you can use those questions in your daily testing and revising. You can record your answers. You will become more fluent and articulate by talking out loud. It bears repeating: Just don't make the mistake of making those facts into mini-essays when you change facts to questions. It will take too long to record, and you will not want to continue.

CHOOSE YOUR TIME FOR TESTING

You know you need to study in the mornings on your days off. But what are the steps you need to take to accommodate the new testing program?

Ensure you have an uninterrupted hour where you can test yourself under exam conditions at home. Test at night for an hour or so (depending on the exam components), right after a full day of work. Here is an example of what you might cover in that hour:

- 30 multiple-choice questions in 25 minutes
- one short-answer question in nine minutes instead of 10
- recording of five or six active reading questions in 15 minutes.

This would be the complete testing session. Find a time when you can do it. Not at 11 pm; earlier in the evening if you can.

That can be a challenge if you have young children. I suggest noise-cancelling headphones for your testing, after you arrange for your partner to look after the children. If you normally bathe the kids and then have dinner right after work, figure out how to accommodate that and still do your testing. Some doctors stay back at work for an extra hour, and then come home. Others have dinner, get the children into bed and then do the testing. Whatever works for you.

Test when you can, but don't use the mornings for this except when you are on night shifts. You may get home around 9 am. Test after you have eaten but before you go to bed. If your days off are limited because you are on call, squeeze in more time for testing before work. You need to be more flexible and adapt your hours when you are on call.

As you get closer to the exam, you need to be selfish. You need to focus more on the exam in the last few weeks before the exam; life is not balanced.

I worked with a senior registrar who was formerly a consultant in his country. He had to redo his Fellowship exams to practise in Australia. He had failed twice. He told me that each time his exams came close, his in-laws would come over to help mind the children. They stayed in the house with the family. Not only that, his study was the guest bedroom and he had to share his study with the in-laws. Also, they were celebrating with friends and other members of the family many nights of the week. The in-laws would make wonderful meals and invite friends and other relatives to come and visit. He couldn't concentrate on his study; people would come and interrupt, "Oh come and have dinner," or, "Would you like a drink?"

I was horrified. I said, "Look, you can't do this. How about you move to a motel by yourself for the last few weeks." He did, and he passed. From then on, he could enjoy visits from the in-laws. They meant well but did not understand. This happens so often. People who are not in medicine do not always understand how difficult the process can be to pass exams.

BE BETTER THAN YOU NEED TO BE

Test the various written components of any exam under speed-versus-accuracy conditions. I've mentioned doing 10-minute short-answer questions in nine minutes. Some surgeons have six-minute questions. Do them in five.

> This encourages your brain to access material and respond more quickly.

Exams are always under time pressure. Often, people fall behind as they go through each question on their exams. Sometimes they spend longer on a question they don't know, but more often they spend extra time on a question they know well, hoping they'll get more marks. They then find they have only a few more minutes for the last few questions and consequently fail. Time management can be an issue.

I used to see a psychiatric trainee who always wrote too much. At the first sitting he didn't finish his written exam and failed. He wrote too much on at least two questions, hoping to get top marks, and then he didn't have time for the others. I had to get him to change the way he worked. It was difficult. He always tweaked what I gave him. He didn't do his homework. He was charming, and talked a lot, usually about golf. Eventually, I suggested to him that he was wasting his time with me unless he listened more carefully and made some of the suggested changes.

He came back eighteen months later, after he'd failed the written exams twice more. He'd made up his mind that maybe some of those strategies could work. To be honest, I think he only came back because he became fed up with consultants telling him he needed to see someone. My primary focus with him was to teach time management strategies for testing each of the exam components, because otherwise there was no way he would complete the exam in the time allocated. He gradually became more concise. Eventually he passed.

MONITOR YOUR PROGRESS

Note how well you do in your diary. Within a few weeks, you will see an improvement. This will increase your confidence. I always give my clients some "homework" at our first session. I see them again in three or four weeks and follow up on how they have managed. By that time, if they have done the work, they notice the difference.

Give your completed short-answer questions, done under test conditions at home, to your supervising consultants at work. Tell them you have done these questions under time restrictions. Consultants would prefer that, rather than a perfect answer written in unrestricted time. They will give you valuable feedback on content and organisation of your responses. If you do test daily, you'll have at least seven completed questions a week, so spread the "joy" of evaluating the questions to a variety of consultants.

You will find answers to MCQs in "black bank" and regular databases. Mark your answers straight away and note down the percentage you get right in your diary. Examiners tell me that if you get about 90% right using the MCQ databases, then you have a good chance of passing the MCQ component.

In terms of oral exams, ask some of your colleagues if they notice a difference in the way you respond to questions. Sometimes, without prompting, colleagues will say, "Gee, you are sounding a bit better." You might even start to be aware of your own increased confidence and your ability to be more fluent when you listen to recordings of yourself.

TEST YOUR KNOWLEDGE OF TESTING

What did you learn in this chapter? Did you read it actively, making a note of any facts and turning those facts into questions to test yourself later?

ACTION PLAN

✓ Practise exam components in shorter time than allowed.
  e.g. 10-minute SAQs in 9 minutes, 5-minute SAQs in 4 minutes.

✓ Get written SAQs marked.

✓ Practise "normal" MCQs under exam conditions.
  e.g. 30x MCQs in 25 minutes.

✓ Record % of correct MCQ answers in your diary – read up on wrong answers in study time.

✓ Record responses to written and/or oral questions.

✓ Verbally describe images, x-rays etc. and record your responses.

✓ Listen and evaluate all your recorded responses from 1 to 10, first for content only, then for voice tone.

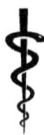

CHAPTER SEVEN

IN ORAL EXAMS, WORDS AREN'T EVERYTHING

"Not everything that can be counted counts,
and not everything that counts can be counted."

ALBERT EINSTEIN

Much of our communication comes through non-verbal communication. Understanding a little about how to use body language and the voice can mean the difference between success and failure. By using non-verbal communication, you can make your responses more authentic and engage the listener.

In this chapter, I'll outline how to improve your non-verbal communications skills, including how often to practise, how to improve your vocal tone, your posture and body language, and how to manage your energy and recover from a distraction to get back on track. With learning, repetition and practice you will develop a response pattern that is automatic and effective.

Albert Mehrabian has become known best by his publications on the relative importance of verbal and non-verbal messages. His initial research back in 1967 suggested that the combined effect of simultaneous verbal, vocal and facial attitude communications is a weighted sum of their independent effects, with the coefficients of .07, .38, and .55, respectively. These figures have been misinterpreted, and it has been widely misquoted around the world that over 90 per cent of communication is nonverbal, with 55 per cent being body language, 38 per cent being the tone of the voice, and only seven per cent relating to the words themselves. I have been guilty of misquoting these figures myself.

However, it is important to recognise that much of our communication comes through non-verbal communication. In fact, if we can't see and hear the non-verbals, then it is easier to misunderstand the words. Think how often we misunderstand emailed communications, or attribute emotions to the words we read. Also, when we are unsure what the words mean, we pay more attention to the non-verbals. This has ramifications in a situation where there is an examiner evaluating your responses. It is generally understood that voice tone and body language are harder to control than words. If you are not very sure about the correctness of your response, then the examiner may pay more attention to your non-verbal communication. Why? So that they can check out the alignment between words, voice and body.

Sometimes we misinterpret signals because of cultural differences. Remember Ali, an emergency registrar mentioned in Chapter 3, who always said yes to overtime requests? The person doing the rosters probably unconsciously observed Ali's compliant body language and would therefore ask Ali first, because there was a good chance he would not refuse to do the overtime.

What I mean by non-verbal communication refers, first, to body language. It is a means of transmitting information, just like the spoken word, except that it is achieved through physical movements, touching, gestures, facial expressions, posture, and even the way you adorn your body through clothes, hairstyle, jewellery, tattoos, etc.

Non-verbal communication also includes voice tone, which refers to how the words sound, not just what is said. People make judgments about others by the way they speak. Voices are flexible, and one can speak with passion, with authority, with humour. But often our voices, either when being evaluated or when speaking in public, become restricted, quiet and monotonous, because of nerves and muscle tightening. Taking control of how your voice is perceived is critical when speaking publicly or when being evaluated.

To master the skill of communication, you need a video and/or voice recorder, so you can monitor yourself on a regular basis. It's easy to use the voice recorder on your smart phone, but with a little practice, you can also use the built-in video recorder as well. Ask a willing partner or friend to help you. They can shoot the video and can let you know if you look like you are struggling. They will be able to give helpful feedback on the way your voice sounds and your overall body language.

Be prepared at first to dislike how you look and sound. Most of us dislike the sound of our recorded voice; and seeing ourselves on video can be excruciating. We tend to be very harsh on the way we look and speak. You will start to notice all the little tics and fidgets that undermine a confident presentation of the facts. However, once you understand this evidence-based approach to non-verbal communication, you can tweak your voice and posture to appear more confident and engage your listener. It is not as hard as you might think.

You must practise daily for confident body language and voice control to become natural.

Your focus should always be on your response and on being authentic. Monitor yourself daily by recording yourself at work, then listening to yourself at home and scoring yourself in your diary. It won't be long before you notice, in work situations and with your family, that people are giving you positive feedback.

DAILY PRACTICE

Read, understand and practise non-verbal communication every day. Doing so will help you shift your focus away from how you feel to responding accurately to the questions and your answers. You will learn to engage the listener more.

A general surgery registrar came to see me a few years back, saying she had lost her self-confidence. She didn't feel listened to or valued. I noticed she slouched and spoke quietly. We worked for much of the hour on making her voice louder. To help her speak louder, I suggested she sit with her shoulders back and breathe in more deeply before speaking. With the increased volume in her voice she sounded more confident. She promised to practise this and made a booking to see me again three weeks later. I was surprised and impressed at the difference in her demeanour. Her posture was better, she spoke in a louder voice, and I didn't have to strain to hear her. I thought she sounded confident and competent. She reported that she now spoke up in her department when she had something to say. Colleagues listened to her, instead of over-riding her soft-spoken comments, and she felt more valued.

The homework I had given this surgery registrar was to practise speaking louder when talking with colleagues in the hospital. She was to remind herself of this by setting an interval timer or her smart phone to vibrate or beep every 30 minutes. It was certainly effective, and soon she did not need to remind herself. It had become second nature.

You can practise better posture in the same way. Consciously straighten your back, pull your shoulders back and lift your head up. Think of a thumbtack pressed firmly between your shoulder blades – ouch! Works every time! Again, set a timer to remind you to concentrate on your posture in your working environment, this will enable you to make effective change. Make the increments from maybe half an hour daily, to an hour, or longer, until you have better posture all the time. By then, your good posture will have become a habit.

In both instances, whether working on having a confident voice or better posture, always monitor yourself daily by giving yourself a score out of 10 and recording it in a diary. The score could be for effectiveness, whether other people noticed a difference, or how long you were able to sustain good posture. The mere action of recording your progress daily will increase your motivation to persist on making improvements.

WHAT'S THE MATTER WITH THE WAY I SPEAK?

According to Toastmaster International, your voice is the primary link between you and your listeners. It is the medium of your message. They say it is most likely that the voice you are now using is not your best voice. You may have buried your optimum speaking voice under layers of bad

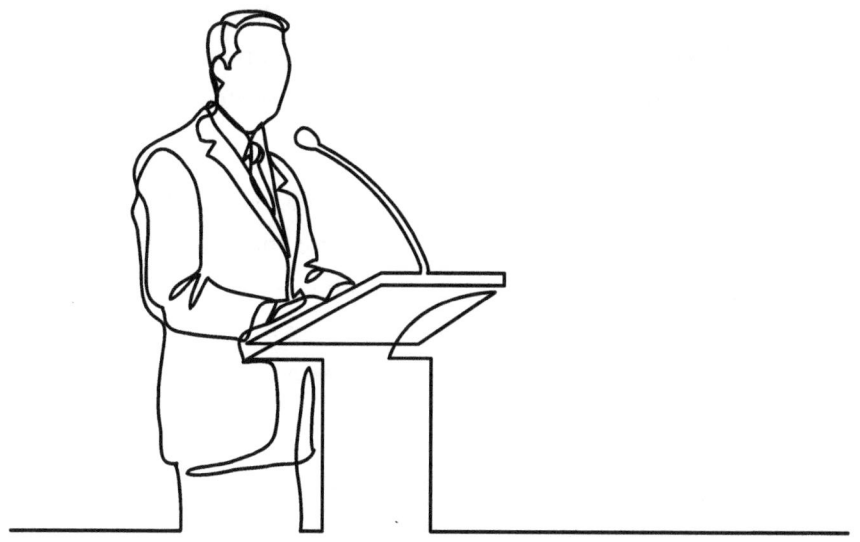

speech habits. In Toastmaster's 2011 article, 'Your Speaking Voice', they state that the voice mirrors your personality with a language all its own – that a natural voice which projects friendliness and authority is a significant tool for personal success.

Think about it! When you speak, your voice reflects your psychological and emotional state of mind. If you are terrified when you are being questioned by examiners, you may have difficulty in persuading or influencing them with your message – or even getting them to listen in a positive way. A natural voice, minus those bad speech habits, engages the listener. It can help you win the respect of others. There are several elements that determine the tone of your voice. According to various authorities these vary between four and twelve elements. I regularly mention the use of voice elements in my practice preparing doctors for oral exams or interviews. The five voice elements that I suggest you consider when listening to your recorded voice are volume, pitch, resonance, diction, pace and pause:

Volume: Correlates to how you breathe. Deep, controlled breathing is necessary for good vocal production. When you breathe in, the abdominal wall expands, and the diaphragm flattens. When you exhale, the diaphragm relaxes and pushes air out of the lungs. The exhaled air provides the controlled production of speech sounds, and volume can be increased. Volume creates a feeling of confidence in your listener and they see you as an authority.

Pitch: This is the up-and-down way you use your voice. It creates interest. Many people talk at a pitch that is too high for them. The high-pitched voice can lack authority and appeal. If you feel your natural pitch could be a bit lower, work on it by consciously pitching your voice slightly lower in all conversation. Maybe just half a tone lower is all that is necessary.

Resonance: This is the opening up of the throat, so you can round out the vowels more readily. The greater resonance we have, the more our listener believes what we say. Radio announcers and TV announcers tend to have good resonance, but if you speak with a nasally twang, as a lot of Australians do, you can sound less believable.

Diction is the fourth voice element. It is controlled when you use the small muscles of the lips, the tongue and the mouth to enunciate each syllable of every word. It improves the clarity with which you speak. We often mumble when we are not sure that what we are saying is correct – a habit that needs to be changed.

Pace and pause is the fifth element. I treat them as one element because they are so closely linked. Pace is the speed at which you speak, and pause is when you stop speaking, usually at the end of a sentence. When we are nervous, we often speak too fast and we do not pause enough. There is a balance between speaking too fast, and too slowly. If we speak a bit slower, it is easier for others to understand us. When you pause, for example at the end of a sentence after making a good point, it allows your listener (the examiner) to comprehend and digest what you have said. Too often doctors being evaluated in an exam will feel they have to rush because there is a time limit in each viva. But what happens is that the examiner may well miss any good points that you are making.

When you listen back to your voice, you will learn to recognise the voice elements you need to change. Select a couple of elements you would like to alter and monitor your recordings daily. Perhaps work on just one element at a time, for instance, volume.

A few years ago, Raji, an intensivist, saw me for a few sessions. He told me that he had learned to speak rapidly without any pauses, and he indicated that it was the way most people he knew had been taught when they learned the English language. At the time I had just read a research article on "power posing" and the effects of testosterone. I thought I would try it out with Raji without telling him what I was doing. I asked him to lean back and place his arms along the back of the sofa. I also asked him to stretch his legs out in a comfortable position and keep talking for a few minutes. I had read that changing the position of the body into a larger position would allow more testosterone to be excreted from the endocrine system. After about 30 seconds Raji interrupted himself and said:

"Patsy, I don't like this. You are my teacher and it is disrespectful to sit like this".

I said, "Raji, just stay like that, I'll explain later."

I had intended to keep Raji in that position for only three or four minutes. However, we were engrossed in conversation and I forgot to tell him to sit normally. After about 20 minutes I noticed he was speaking a little slower and the pitch of his voice had gone down just a fraction. I thought to myself, "Goodness, he's starting to sound like a consultant." Then I suddenly remembered that I'd forgotten to change him back to his normal sitting position. As I opened my mouth to say something, he said:

"You know, Patsy, I really rather like sitting like this. I feel pretty good."

I explained what I had done.

He said, "Oh, I am going to practise this every day until the exam."

The exam was about three weeks away. He passed, and I'd like to think that it was in part because his voice was a little slower and deeper, and he used more confident body language.

BODY LANGUAGE

SUCCESS STORY

A few months ago, a general practitioner told me he could not get through his orals. I saw immediately what was happening. As he talked to me, he wiggled. He pulled faces when I asked him a question. I pointed out to him what he was doing. He was astonished. I asked him to practise at home with his wife observing his movements. He was to try and sit still and keep his

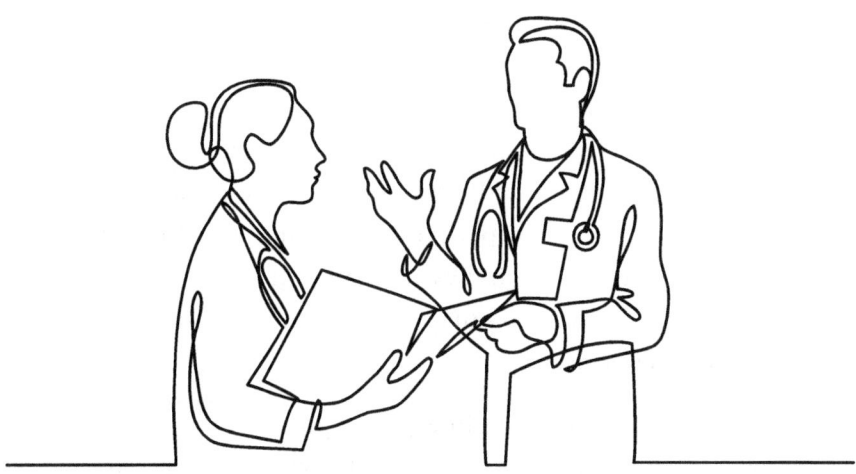

face more composed while answering questions. What an improvement at the next visit. He sat perfectly still, using only one hand to gesticulate. He spoke clearly without pulling faces. He handled himself much better in the oral exam.

As mentioned earlier, body language is a group of behaviours including gestures, posture and facial expressions. Observe yourself in the mirror or get your partner or friend to observe or video you as you answer an oral question. You can see what needs to change. Change only happens with self-awareness. It's useful to ask your partner or friend to suggest what needs fixing as you're talking. For instance, your hands may flail around. Perhaps you pull a face or roll your eyes as you think of a response. Perhaps you wriggle or put your hand up near your mouth when you're less than confident about your answer. Maybe you scratch your nose, or your body sways from side to side.

POWER POSTURES

Research on the effects of testosterone was carried out on a colony of chimpanzees by social psychologist Amy Cuddy and colleagues a few years ago. It was found that the alpha male had high testosterone (a dominance hormone), and low cortisol (a stress hormone), and the rest of the colony had high cortisol and low testosterone. When the alpha male was deposed, the new alpha male almost immediately had high testosterone and low cortisol. Cuddy's research questions were: Does this happen with humans, and if so, how long does it take? In a study carried out on human participants it was found that it does occur, and it can take three or four minutes to change from increased cortisol to increased testosterone by enlarging the body's position. This was referred to as "power posing".

As the story about Raji sitting in a power pose suggests, it is possible to decrease or increase testosterone and cortisol by the posture you assume. If you tend to cross your arms and legs and maintain a small position, the chances are that you increase the amount of cortisol in your system and you don't feel powerful. However, if you maintain a big body position – shoulders back, head up, arms by the side or akimbo, and legs outstretched, then you are more likely to increase the amount of testosterone in your system and you feel powerful. Cuddy's work has since been criticised, but analysis over many studies on body language clearly demonstrates a link between expansive postures and feelings of power. Those in high power poses feel more powerful than their low-pose counterparts and are perceived to be more confident. Reflect on the way different high-status people walk around. Think of the consultant surgeon striding through the hospital corridors, or the principal of a school strolling around the playground, or even a couple of police officers walking along their beat. If you look closely you will notice that the head is up, their shoulders are back, the hands are behind their back or at their sides. They may not know it, but they are subconsciously exhibiting a lack of fear. How does one know? They are not protecting the most vulnerable parts of a human body – the throat, the chest, and the stomach.

Doctors who are sitting oral exams would really benefit from feeling more powerful while being evaluated. Because it takes such a short time (three minutes or so) to increase the level of testosterone, it could be done while waiting in the corridor before an interview. Perhaps while reading instructions or a clinical scenario before entering the exam room for a cross-table viva. One could even "power pose" while in the restroom!

SUCCESS STORY

A doctor emailed me after her exam performance. I had previously talked about power posing while she was having consultations with me and had suggested she use it wherever possible. She said in her email, "The superwoman body stance was incredible. I started doing it in the privacy of a bathroom cubicle but by the second day of the exam, I was standing like this in the holding bay where they kept us in the 15 minutes leading up to the examination. I did it for five minutes at least every time.

"I was there with six candidates cooped up at a time in a tiny corridor, waiting for the group beforehand to finish. You could have cut the tension with a knife. I noticed the other candidates with me (they all happened to be males) would stand with their hands in their pockets head down or they were leaning over sitting down with their spread legs and the head down. I disengaged myself from any conversation and instead focused on standing in superwoman posture, looking up, staring out the window at the gently swaying leaves on the tree or at a painting of fishes hanging on the wall. Combined with the deep breathing, it instilled in me a sense of calm. So, when we eventually got called, I stepped forth with confidence and purpose."

ENERGY REGULATION REVISITED

In Chapter 5 we looked at energy regulation from the point of view of lowering your body activation and thus increasing your focus to the task. I pointed out that a diaphragmatic breath such as the centering breath would be useful for performing difficult procedures, or as part of a pre-performance routine for written questions.

Energy regulation also affects how other people perceive you, which means it is a vital part of your communication with others.

Alex was an ear, nose and throat registrar, who was sitting his Fellowship exam for the first time. He told me that he was being grilled almost daily by consultants. He said that when he knew the answers to questions he answered immediately with no initial pause, and his voice was confident. Consultants were satisfied with his answers. However, when he wasn't quite sure of himself, even if he gave the right answer, consultants would know almost instantly. When I asked how they would know, Alex said it was because he paused for a while before answering and his eyes would dart around while searching for the answer. Consultants would then ask more questions because the messages they received from his non-verbal communication were incongruent with what might have been the correct answers.

The key here was that Alex replied quickly when he was confident of his answer and was more hesitant to start his answer when he wasn't sure. By teaching Alex how and when to use the centering breath, not only before the questions he was doubtful about, but also before the questions he knew well, the consultants wouldn't observe such obvious clues that he was unsure of his answer. It meant that Alex paused in the same way before responding to all questions, even to questions he knew. Once he started doing this he found his eyes didn't dart around as much, as he was calmer and more focused on giving a good response. The centering breath had lowered his body activation. It was not so obvious to consultants that he was trying to think of something to say. It ended up that he wasn't being grilled as rigorously as before.

The secret to acing your exams is to stay calm under pressure. After all, taking a big breath helps to integrate body and mind. Recognise when you need to sequence the centering breath you were taught in Chapter 5. Awareness of personal stress points makes your ability to plan where you want to take a breath much easier. Sequencing refers to planning where, based on previous experience, you know you are likely to have increased body activation during your written and oral exams, and you plan to take a centering breath at those times. You know when to put them in. Try to take a centering breath before answering a consultant, as it stops you blurting out the beginning of an answer, and then digging a hole for yourself. List what always makes you nervous about answering questions. For instance, does an examiner who is poker-faced or disdainful make you nervous. Do you struggle to think of the right word if the examiner asks you, "Are you sure?" or prompts you with a question such as "Anything else?" So, practise taking a breath before answering a question so that you can regain your focus.

SUCCESS STORY

Recently, a registrar came to me upset after failing an oral exam a few months earlier. She thought the examiner looked at her disdainfully. She felt stupid, became anxious and couldn't answer the questions properly. I suggested she find a friendly consultant and ask that person to look disdainfully at her when she answered questions in the lead-up to the next exam. She laughed at my suggestion, but she followed my advice and found a consultant who was happy to help. She practised several times and found she became immune to consultants who made faces or looked haughty. Everyone is affected by body language. Don't allow examiners' approval or disapproval to affect your performance.

HINTS TO REGAIN FOCUS AFTER DISTRACTION

No matter how well you prepare for your exams and practise communication skills, you can lose focus. Everyone does. A thought pops into your head, and it distracts you. The examiner appears unfriendly. Somebody sneezes or a door slams shut. Anything can happen which may distract you.

> ## The difference between those who pass and those who fail is the ability to recover from distraction and re-focus.

Learning and practising, making lots of errors, is part of the learning process. Eventually, after enough repetitious re-focusing, your ability to overcome distractions will improve dramatically. You will be able to smoothly regain focus. This leads to "automaticity", which is the ability to do things without occupying the mind with the low-level details required. With learning, repetition and practice you develop an automatic response pattern or habit. Practise enough at home and at work, then under exam conditions you are more likely to regain focus on your responses to questions.

Here are some ways to regain focus:

- Use the centering breath.
- Use a muscle relaxation technique that relaxes your shoulders, which your examiner will not notice. There's a sitting and a standing version:
  Sitting – grip your hands under the chair base and pull up hard for three or four seconds without lifting your shoulders. Build the tension and then relax. Your shoulders will relax.
  Standing – push your thumb and first finger together for three to four seconds. Push hard and then release. Again, your shoulders will relax.
- Look at the examiner's third eye – the space between their eyebrows. Because your focus softens, you don't become

distracted by all the micro expressions on the examiner's face. You no longer see all the little muscles surrounding the eyes of the examiner, yet the examiner will feel they have eye contact with you. Many candidates in exams react to those facial expressions and change their answers. Examiners are trained to try and keep a blank expression, but that is hard to do. And even a blank expression can be unsettling to some people. If you look at the space between their eyebrows, you will block out those micro facial expressions.

PUT IT ALL TOGETHER TO IMPROVE YOUR COMMUNICATION SKILLS

Each of these steps increases your ability to engage in good non-verbal communication. As your skills improve, the positive reactions you get from others at work and home will be a reward in itself. Think about the difference between a real patient scenario in the hospital and the exam-based scenario. You probably don't have these non-verbal communication problems when you are with a patient because the focus is not on you, but on your patient's care. You are more dynamic, more authentic in the way you sound. Try to have the same mindset in an exam. Pretend it is a handover, that you are going away and want to impart everything you know to the person taking over your case.

A critic of my approach might say that all you need to do is answer the question and you will pass. The research is against them. Our responses to non-verbal communication are instinctive and beyond our control. Even if your examiner wanted to ignore your body language and vocal tone, they could not. You will lose points because of poor non-verbal communication.

ACTION PLAN

✓ Monitor your body language on video – get partner or friend to also give feedback.

✓ Ascertain which of the five voice elements you need to improve.

✓ Set an interval timer to vibrate every 30 minutes to remind you of body posture and voice tone.

✓ Monitor yourself daily on some aspect of body language or voice elements.

✓ Keep your shoulders back and head up when responding to consultants – monitor daily.

✓ Use the centering breath before responding to consultants' questions to stay focused.

✓ List when you might need to use the centering breath – everybody is different.

✓ Ask a friendly consultant to act in a way you don't like when responding to questions.

✓ Use a sitting or standing muscle relaxation technique to refocus.

✓ Look at space between eyebrows of examiner when responding to questions.

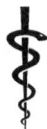

CHAPTER EIGHT

HABITS – WHEN WILLPOWER IS WASTED

*"Good habits are as addictive as bad habits,
and a lot more rewarding."*

HARVEY MACKAY

This chapter is all about developing habits – good habits – that will save you from the exhaustion of using willpower to get your study done. When you develop good study habits, you will free yourself from procrastination and self-sabotaging thoughts. Your brain won't be working overtime and worrying won't be such a problem. Eventually any bad habits that are neglected, will disappear. You will learn to break down your goals into simple tasks, develop insight into your behaviour, and persist after relapses.

Every day, in one form or another, you exert willpower. You resist the urge to look at emails instead of studying. You reach for a salad when you really want a cake. You bite your tongue when you'd like to make a snide remark. Yet research indicates that resisting repeated temptations takes a mental toll. Willpower is like a muscle that can get fatigued from overuse. If you rely on willpower to study every day, you will probably fall by the wayside.

Practise anything consistently every day and you will create habits. Think about that morning coffee you just can't do without. It's a habit. Try this little exercise. Just cross your arms in front of your body. Feels comfortable, doesn't it? Now reverse the position of your arms and cross them the other way. It feels awkward, doesn't it? Yet, if you persisted in always crossing your arms this way for about two or three weeks, it would no longer be awkward – you would have created a new habit. But do you want to cross your arms differently? Probably not.

Well-known author and educator Stephen Covey defines a habit as "the intersection of knowledge, skill and desire". He explains that knowledge is **what** to do, skill is **how** to do it, and desire is the **want** to do it. For instance, you might have the *knowledge* to respond to a consultant's question with the correct answer, even though it took about 100 words instead of 10. The *skill* is to make your answer succinct and clear. The *desire* is having the motivation to practise and make that change.

Be prepared to use self-discipline at first, and bravely face change. Relapses may happen. Persist and, over time, new and positive habits will emerge. After a while an activity of this type becomes autonomous, but this relies on you being diligent with daily practice. We need to be aware of our mistakes while practising – correct them straight away and learn from them. It is sometimes too easy to let a mistake go, maybe thinking "I'll do better tomorrow." For example, if you listened on the same day to a recorded response to a consultant's question and you cringed at the way you answered, then while it is still fresh, re-record a response, correcting some of those errors. This is an effective way to learn from mistakes. According to Stephen Covey "the power to make and keep commitments to ourselves is the essence of developing the basic habits of effectiveness."

Monitor your activities in your diary. You will feel an increased sense of wellbeing, and a sense that your life is falling into place. If you want to read the definitive book on habits, try Stephen Covey's *The 7 Habits of*

Highly Effective People. He explains how developing good habits leads to increased wellbeing and happy, successful people, rather than driven people who succeed in the narrow sense of the word.

In the meantime, you can get started with the following information about stages of learning, change, procrastination and sabotaging thoughts.

THREE STAGES OF LEARNING

Way back in 1967 a three-stage learning model was presented by Fitts and Posner. To this day it is still considered applicable for motor learning. As a sport and exercise psychologist I have used this model of learning over the years for a variety of activities. I believe it is appropriate for preparing for written and clinical exams.

1ST STAGE OF LEARNING – THE COGNITIVE STAGE

The first stage is where the learner focuses on cognitive-oriented problems. The learner tries to answer questions such as, "Why should I do my SAQ in nine minutes rather than 10 minutes? How should I vary my pre-performance routine for different exam components? How do I hide my nervousness when I answer verbal questions?" I find that the less experienced the person the more readily they can change. Experienced doctors have been doing it their way most of their working life. They have old habits and find it hard to let go.

But it is easier to teach new habits than to try and fix old habits. One experienced surgeon I worked with used beta blockers to deal with his anxiety prior to departmental presentations. It wasn't always effective, as he couldn't quite get the dose right. He would sometimes be talking to an audience and be aware of his heart beating loudly and slowly. He found it very distracting. Rather than fiddle around with the dose to get it right, I persuaded him to use a breathing technique to lower his heart rate, so that he could better control his body activation. It took a while for him to have the courage to use this breathing technique regularly, as he had learned to rely on beta blockers.

This stage of learning a new skill takes lots of practice, and it is normal to have lots of errors. The way to learn is from your mistakes - which gradually decrease over time - until you reach the next stage.

2ND STAGE OF LEARNING – THE ASSOCIATIVE STAGE

The transition into this stage occurs after lots of practice, when the trainee knows what, when, and how to do the different tasks associated with good study and testing for the written and clinical exams. For instance, if you learn the centering technique (Chapter 5) and practise it a lot, you develop knowledge of what it's used for (perhaps before reading or answering a question), why to do it (so it lowers the heart rate and allows for increased focus on a question), and the motivation to want to practise it. There are fewer mistakes at this stage, but doing the skill still requires a conscious effort, or concentration. However, through over-learning and lots of practice, the repetitive actions become more habitual, which leads to the final stage.

3RD STAGE OF LEARNING – AUTONOMOUS

The third stage is when the skill becomes effortless. No longer does the trainee have to think about when, where and how to study, or to take a deep breath, or to record and listen to their responses. By this time the trainee has had so much repetitive practice that their studying and testing has become second nature. Little thinking is involved. Over time these skills have required less conscious attention and effort and can be performed quicker. They have become automatic or habitual. Habits form when there is repetitious behaviour such as over-learning and practice.

Let's take the example of the centering breath. In the second stage of learning, remembering to take a breath at the appropriate time requires a conscious effort. With practice, the centering breath becomes automatic. When you feel your body beginning to activate, for whatever reason, you automatically take a breath and feel calmer and more focused. You also are aware of situations where you would expect to feel nervous, such as being grilled by a consultant during a handover or being watched while doing a difficult procedure. In these circumstances you now automatically take a breath beforehand, and the stress is lessened.

REPETITIOUS ACTIVITIES LEAD TO HABITS

Habits are different from willpower, where you actively control or steer your choices. Willpower comes and goes depending on how much you've already used that day. Willpower is strongest early in the day. If you study in the mornings on tasks you dislike first, you will get them over with.

The tasks you like, which you do later, do not require as much willpower. Evidence suggests that willpower-depleted individuals might be low on "brain fuel". The brain is a high-energy organ, powered by a steady supply of glucose (blood sugar).

Studies have shown that people who exerted willpower in laboratory tasks had lower glucose levels than control subjects who weren't asked to draw on their self-control. Roy Baumeister is a social psychologist who explores how we think about the self, and why we feel and act the way we do. He is especially known for his work on willpower, self-control and self-esteem, and how they relate to success. In one of several studies Baumeister and his colleagues invited participants into a room where the table before them held a bowl of chocolates and a bowl of radishes. Half the participants were invited to eat the chocolates, while the other half were asked to eat only the radishes. No-one stayed in the room to supervise them. Then all the participants were given 30 minutes to complete a difficult geometric puzzle. The participants who ate the radishes (and had to resist the chocolates) gave up on the puzzle after about eight minutes, while the lucky chocolate eaters persevered for almost 19 minutes.

Baumeister concluded that drawing on willpower to resist the chocolates drained people's self-control in facing subsequent challenges. You will face this challenge when you have a morning exam followed by an afternoon exam on the same day. The chances are that you will be tired and flat during the afternoon exam because of the mental effort of doing the morning exam. It means that the lunch break after the morning exam should be devoted to rest and recovery to prepare for the afternoon exam. Too often doctors like to get together over the lunch break and discuss how they went in the morning exam, or they go over their notes in preparation for the afternoon exam. This does not allow the brain to recuperate.

> It's easier on the brain if you have a structure that fosters good habits. There is no need to waste time and energy deciding if you will or won't do something today. You just do it.

IF IT'S BROKE, CHANGE IT

Unless you change whatever it is you are doing, your old patterns will stay the same, and the chances are that you will have difficulty getting through your exams. Change what isn't working for you or it's the same old, same old.

One of my clients, Emily, was a radiation oncologist, a little older than most other trainees. Emily did not seem highly motivated to change her habits despite having failed her written exams a couple of times. At each visit, I offered her some different suggestions to try and motivate within her a desire to change. The next time I saw her, she always had an excuse for not having carried out the activities. She had a busy week. She was too tired. Or she had a wedding, or some other function, which she had promised to attend.

I noticed that Emily went to gym classes regularly and preferred to go on weekend mornings, despite this being an ideal time to study. She explained that she made up for it by studying in the afternoons – if she didn't have other commitments. She had ideal work shifts: days only, with weekends off, so it would have been easy to have had regular study times. At the next session I asked Emily to write down all the reasons why she had not changed her study patterns, always prefacing the reason with the words "I can't". After that was completed, I asked her to read them out to me but changing the words "I can't" with "I won't". For example, "I can't study because I didn't get to bed till late last night", was changed to "I won't study because I didn't get to bed till late last night". This exercise made her thoughtful and quiet. I think she realised that she was in denial and just wasn't doing enough study. I'd like to say there was immediate and outstanding improvement in her attitude towards her study. There wasn't; there was a slight change. Not enough to pass the third time. Eventually Emily did get through, but what a waste of time, and thousands of dollars of exam fees.

Studies of change have found that people move through a series of stages when modifying behaviour. The Transtheoretical Model, developed by Prochaska and DiClemente, in 1983, is based on principles developed from leading theories of counselling and behaviour change. This model is currently in use by professionals around the world, and has five consistent stages:

1. **Pre-contemplative** – a person is not interested in change; can't see the need to change.
2. **Contemplation** – they are starting to think about the issue and the possible need to make some changes.

3. **Preparation** – a change is about to happen because they realise that the situation is serious.
4. **Action** – they have made real and overt changes or modifications and are starting to see the results. Relapse and temptation are still very strong.
5. **Maintenance** – they consolidate changes in behaviour to maintain the new status quo, and previously learned coping strategies are in place to prevent relapse or temptation.

Which stage of change are you at? Be aware of all the times you say, "I can't"." I can't do four hours of study each morning on my day off. I can't get up in the morning." Or "I can't do an hour's test every night. I'm too tired." Change that word "can't" to "won't". You will find this changes your perception. If you are failing your exams, what you are doing is not working for you. You need to change what you are doing. Go back and look at your answers to the questionnaire at the end of Chapter 1.

RECOGNISE PROCRASTINATION

Procrastinators have a common justification for putting off till tomorrow what they could do today: they believe they perform better under pressure, when it's so close to the deadline that they will just have to do the work. How did you answer those questions in Chapter 2?

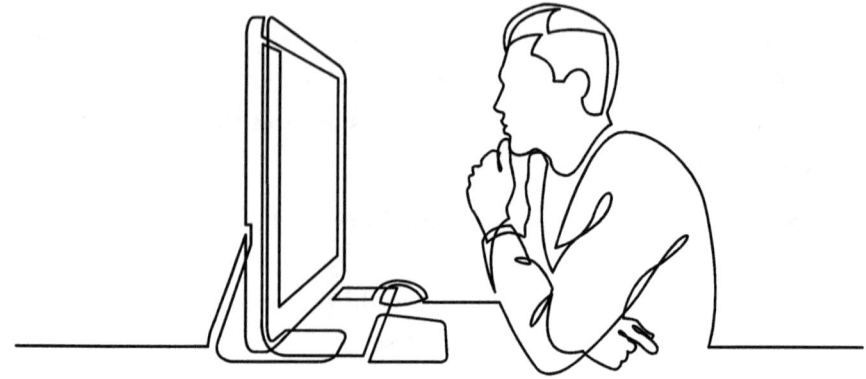

It is most unusual for people to perform better under pressure unless they do the preparation. Think about some of the most pressured professionals in the world: rock-climbers, for example, or cave divers, or soldiers. They don't leave their preparation to the last minute because they know procrastinating could cost them their life.

NO PLAN, NO WAY

This book provides you with a concrete plan. It's based on evidence and science and my experience with many hundreds of doctors who have come before you. If you don't have a good well-thought-out plan, you are more likely to procrastinate.

YOU WON'T FEEL BETTER TOMORROW

Learn to recognise that you can have negative emotions without acting on them. You are procrastinating if you say, "I'll feel more like study tomorrow." Acknowledge that the negative emotions you feel today will be worse tomorrow, unless you get started, anyway.

Procrastination is exhausting.

We only have a finite amount of willpower each day, as research by Roy Baumeister and his colleagues have repeatedly found. An effort of will or self-control is tiring. If you are tired all the time, in addition to the long hours you work, it is also because you are forcing yourself to study. Because you don't have good habits, you are less willing or less able to exert self-control when the next challenge comes around.

I must admit I'm a bit of a procrastinator at times. Some tasks I don't like doing. However, I've improved over the years because I teach my clients about avoiding procrastination. I learned how to deal with their obstacles by dealing with my own.

One thing I've always hated doing is putting out the garbage and recycling bins the night before pickup. I don't want to leave my computer or my favourite TV show to go outside and wrestle those dirty, smelly bins onto the footpath. I keep saying to myself, "I'll do it at the next ad break", or "I'll finish this paragraph first". I would use up all my energy reminding myself to put the garbage out. Then I'd forget completely.

What often happened then is that at 6 am, while sipping my morning coffee, I'd suddenly hear a garbage truck turning the corner into my street. I'd hear the crash of bottles emptied into the truck, or the barking of local dogs as the truck proceeded down the laneway. In my pyjamas, with hair all messed up, bleary-eyed, and looking very dishevelled, I'd rush to my garage, open the door, grab my bins to try and have them outside and ready for pickup. More often than I care to admit, I had to chase the truck down the street hauling a bin or two and feeling really embarrassed.

Now, as soon as the thought pops into my head that it's garbage night, I say to myself "Just do it, Patsy". I stop whatever I'm doing immediately and put the garbage out. It works!

TOO MANY UNCERTAINTIES AND DISTRACTIONS

We're most likely to procrastinate on tasks that lack structure. Your concrete plan must be broken down into well-defined steps. If you think too much when you sit down to study, you are likely to procrastinate. If you are uncertain about how to proceed, you haven't planned well and are likely to procrastinate.

If you are distracted, you are procrastinating. Turn off the email, put your phone on silent, isolate yourself as much as you can before you start studying. You are procrastinating if the environment around you is undermining your efforts rather than strengthening your new habits and increased focus of attention.

Jenny came to see me because she was so anxious and distracted before speaking. She gave weekly presentations to consultants and was so nervous that her performance was suffering. She was relaxed talking with patients and their families but felt, incorrectly, that her colleagues and consultants negatively evaluated her all the time.

I explained to her that fear is driven by a complex process in the brain. As I outlined earlier in this book, fear is picked up in your amygdala, which responds to threats almost half a second before you consciously perceive the threat. Your body is primed for fight or flight. Your senses are heightened so you can respond quickly; it is a shortcut that allows your body to react to threat and get you to safety. This quick response was very useful for evolutionary purposes, but we no longer have life and death situations much of the time. We don't want to be constantly in a state of fight or flight. It's not good for our health and increases our stress levels.

However, we can control this. I told Jenny that when she became aware that her body was activated, and her senses were heightened, then the prefrontal cortex – the decision-making area of the brain – could calm down the amygdala. Remember my analogy of the amygdala being a horse that spooks easily, and the prefrontal cortex an expert rider who has techniques to soothe the horse? This analogy resonated with Jenny and she was keen to learn some breathing and thought-stopping techniques. These, with practice, were useful, and she was more able to present material to hospital staff without extreme fear disabling her.

SABOTAGING THOUGHTS WILL ... SABOTAGE YOU

Avoid vacillating about whether to study or not – thoughts can sabotage your plans. Follow the advertising slogan of the shoe-maker, Nike: "Just do it". (As a matter of interest this phrase was inspired by the final words of a criminal who was asked if he had any last thoughts before he faced death by firing squad in 1976.)

SUCCESS STORY

I remember seeing a young executive, Ralph, who was losing his self-confidence because of sabotaging thoughts. He had been promoted from a line manager to a global executive. He was young and bright, but lacked confidence about his new job, particularly when he was asked to present his ideas at regular board meetings. All the other executives were older and more experienced than him. When he was sitting in at the board meetings waiting to present his material, his mind was full of sabotaging thoughts. "They know so much more than me". "I feel like an imposter". "What if I can't answer their questions?" "I shouldn't be here. I'm not good enough."

When Ralph told me that he usually had a couple of cups of strong coffee before each weekly board meeting, I guessed that probably he was up the night before preparing for the meeting. He agreed and said he needed the coffee to stay focused. Since the board meetings were mid-week, Ralph would prepare his talks at night after a full day's work. He found he struggled to be creative and couldn't remember the material he covered at night when he made the presentation. He also said that he would finish off his presentation by about midnight, but then would toss and turn for several hours before finally sleeping.

My first suggestion was that he spend an hour or two in the early mornings before work getting his material ready, as that would be when he was fresh. As discussed in Chapter 3, research indicates that the brain is most active in the morning after a good night's sleep, and thus absorbs and retains information more easily. My second suggestion was that when he needed to do the final preparation for his presentation the night before, that he wore orange-coloured glasses while sitting at his computer. Melatonin is produced by the pineal gland and regulates our sleep and wakefulness. The blue light emitted by devices such as computers, smart phones, and ipads suppresses the body's ability to secrete melatonin, a hormone that makes us sleepy. I suggested to him that the orange lenses would block the melatonin-robbing light coming from his computer. He would then sleep better and be more refreshed on the day of the presentation. My third suggestion was that he record portions of his talk and listen to them to give himself feedback regarding the relevance and quality of the information he was imparting, and how he sounded as he talked.

Ralph took on all these suggestions and changed the way he prepared for presentations at board meetings. Over three weeks or so the change in Ralph was remarkable – he felt more energetic, he remembered more of what he prepared, and consequently he felt more confident at the weekly board meetings. The sabotaging thoughts disappeared.

If you allow yourself to vacillate then there will be a spiral of negative thoughts, many of which are fearful, and this will probably be followed by putting off your study till you feel better.

Repetitious morning study when you're fresh and then testing under fatigue conditions, becomes a habit. It's a little like cleaning your teeth in the morning and evening. I bet you don't consciously think, "Shall I clean my teeth or not?" It has become a ritual, just something you do. There are no self-sabotaging thoughts. That's the way you want your study to be. Make the Nike saying "Just do it" your mantra.

If you "Just do it", you avoid the negative thoughts, guilt and even self-hatred that start to swirl around in your brain when you put off study.

As good habits start to kick in, you will find that those negative thoughts will dissipate, and be replaced by feelings of well-being and self-control.

Over the years, many university students have come to me for advice on their failing grades. One factor that affected their grades was that these students didn't get to their lectures, particularly if they were in the morning. Even more so if it was wintertime. Students weren't necessarily asleep – they just had lots of negative thoughts about getting up and starting the day. One student, Ken, found it so hard to get out of bed that he would put the snooze alarm on time after time. I suggested he put his phone on the other side of the room. He'd roll out of bed, turn the alarm off and stagger back to bed, telling himself he'd get up in a minute or so.

Finally, I asked Ken to get a cheap travel alarm, place it in a tin can and put it over by the door, which was to be left open. He then had to set the alarm on his phone and place it on the other side of the room well away from the travel alarm clock. The phone and the travel alarm were set so that they would go off at the same time. This worked. By having to turn off two alarms at the same time, walking from one side of the room to the other, and with the travel alarm clock reverberating loudly in a tin can, Ken woke up sufficiently to overcome any negative thoughts and avoid the temptation to go back to bed.

He was helped by his flatmates, who didn't appreciate the noise, and yelled for him to get up. Because he was getting up in time to attend lectures, Ken stopped berating himself later. He stopped feeling guilty that he was letting his family down by failing some of his subjects. Without those self-sabotaging thoughts undermining him, he started to have more energy, understood the material presented in lectures, and maintained passing grades.

HABITS SAVE ENERGY AND TIME, AND MAKE YOU SUCCESSFUL

All these steps help to revise the circuitry in the brain so that it is easier to focus your strength, resist temptation and redirect energy. Remember the phrase, 'practice makes perfect'? That is all about changing your brain as you develop your skill.

With better habits, you will increase your sense of satisfaction and wellbeing. Some people might say this is a very rigid approach. But research in neuroscience is increasing our knowledge of the brain.

The brain reacts positively to structure, and works well in short bursts, with recovery in between.

Repetition is how new habits are formed and old habits die for good. We need to change old habits into good habits. Three weeks is often enough time to set a new habit.

ACTION PLAN

✓ Reflect and list old patterns of behaviour you want to change.

✓ Always monitor your behaviours in a diary, noting any improvement.

✓ List some of the things you can't change, and change "can't" to "won't".

✓ Catch yourself procrastinating? Say "Just do it".

✓ Consider programs that reduce the blue light or purchasing orange-tinted glasses for late nights at the computer.

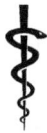

CHAPTER NINE

ELEMENTS OF SUCCESS

"Enthusiasm is a vital element toward the individual success of every man and woman."

CONRAD HILTON

In this brief penultimate chapter, I'd like you to step back and have a look at what else can contribute to your success.

Imagine preparing for the simplest physical competition in the Olympic Games: the 100-metre sprint. I believe there are three elements of success in this event. One is the start. The second is the speed and the length of the stride along the track. The third is the push through beyond the finish line. Those are the elements of success to do well in the 100-metre sprint.

Psychologically, even if we only look at the start, there are certain activities that take place before you get down on the blocks. Just warming up behind the blocks you may find, in a major event, that other sprinters in the race are trying to appear more dominant and confident. They could be strutting around making their warm-up obvious or perhaps making comments. This could be what I call "psyching out".

Maybe there's a little voice in your head distracting you. For instance, it might be saying: "What was my previous time? Gee, I didn't perform well at the last meet? Who is that in the next lane to me? Is it the national champion? Is it somebody I don't know? Are there selectors watching me sprint? Is my partner up in the stands watching?" All these thoughts influence the start of your sprint. This is going to impact on how focused you are when you finally place your feet in the blocks ready to race. The start is the time when you need to focus your senses on listening for the start gun and having an excellent reaction time.

When you think of the elements of success for passing an exam, one of them would, of course, be studying and focusing on understanding the material. Another might be regular testing of exam components. Studying at the optimal time of day for your brain and testing under exam conditions at other times will enhance those elements. You must also look at exercise and nourishment, and when to spend time with your family.

What are the elements of success for your wellbeing and recovery after studying?

You need to maintain your focus on why you want to do this. Your love of medicine? Your desire to achieve excellence? You can sometimes lose that focus, or your reasons for doing the exams, because you are so caught up in the day-to-day business of living. It is a rigorous process to go through the training program and come out the other side. The Fellowship exam is the main barrier to overcome. After that, you get your life back. Often, by the time people come to me, they have forgotten why they want to pass. It has become an ordeal.

There is a quote at the beginning of Chapter One, by Bob Mitchin, which says "The difference between an adventure and an ordeal is attitude."

Reflect on why you want to do this exam. Maybe change your perspective. Make the exam an adventure or a challenge, rather than an ordeal.

PLAN THE DAY

There's one more key element of success, and that's your plan for the big (exam) day.

Many doctors have done all the planning for their study, but contact me before their exams and say, "Right, I want to talk about the day itself. Can you help me?"

I start by asking what time the first exam is and what time they get up.

Some say, "Oh, I roll out of bed at 7 am, the exam is at 8.30."

I say, "No, if the exam is at 8.30, you need to be awake three hours beforehand. You need your body and mind to be warmed up and fully ready to perform."

For about three or four minutes before getting out of bed on the day of the exam, I suggest a little affirmation exercise. I ask doctors to look at the ceiling and physically smile (this smile will lead to positive feelings). They then say to themselves phrases such as: "I'm looking forward to today." "I've worked hard for this." "I'm going to show them what I can do." "This is going to be a good day". "I know a lot of material." Doing this first thing before getting ready to go to the exam venue just takes away that very slight chance that you might get out of bed feeling grumpy and out of sorts and may stay that way all day.

But that's just the beginning of your planning. It's vital that you have every aspect of the exam day meticulously planned. This includes Plan A for how you want things to go, and Plan B, which accounts for potential problems. This will help you feel more in control, have a positive attitude, and focus less on feeling anxious and debilitated.

Here are some things to consider for your Plan A and Plan B.

PLAN A

- Know exactly when your first exam starts, how long you have for a break, and when the next exam begins.
- Plan for travel to the venue so that there's no last-minute panic if there is an accident on the freeway or there are roadworks.
- Decide exactly what you will do after you register at the venue and before the exam starts. I suggest that you close your eyes so you don't get talking to other people who feel anxious. Perhaps do a mindfulness technique (that counting breath mentioned in Chapter 5 would be useful) until the bell goes.
- Plan what you will do in breaks between exams. For example, you might decide to have no post-mortems before the last exam, or you might have glucose on hand before afternoon exams to avoid the mid-afternoon slump. Maybe you could freshen up in the bathroom, to assist recovery and be more alert before the second exam.

PLAN B

- Be prepared for potential problems by having spare pens that write smoothly, or bringing earplugs in case there is a disturbance, such as someone constantly coughing, or having an extra layer of clothing in case the room is too cold.
- If there's a delay between exams, what will you do? Keep occupied. Drink water. Do a centering breath or mindfulness technique. Do some stretching of your shoulders and the neck, or any areas where we hold tension. Circle your shoulders and loosen them up to get rid of tension.

ACTION PLAN

✓ What are the elements essential for focused study?

✓ What are the distractions you need to overcome to be successful in your study program?

✓ List what you would find beneficial to increase your wellbeing and recovery after studying.

✓ Write an outline of your Plan A for the exam day/s and add the details as soon as you know the timetable.

✓ What is your Plan B for those unexpected moments before or during the exam? Be creative!

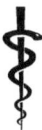

CHAPTER TEN

SELF-BELIEF – SUCCESS IS COOL, AND THIS IS WHY

"My job is to awaken possibility in other people."

BENJAMIN ZANDER

Successful doctors have a high degree of self-confidence, block out distractions, manage their energy levels, and are goal-oriented. The good habits developed through constant repetition of the techniques in this book create self-belief. You start to feel in control, your attitude changes towards your exams, sabotaging thoughts diminish, and life is a little more balanced. You have, over time, developed mental toughness, which is essentially a set of various mental skills such as focus, the ability to perform under pressure, resilience, motivation, and unshakeable self-belief.

When you develop self-belief, you tend to pass exams more readily. You don't chop and change how you do your study, or study in the same old way. You have a more balanced life and feel better – healthier, more connected to friends and family, and much less stressed.

While the needs of each doctor will vary, there are common strategies used by elite performers in many fields. Do as many of the techniques as you think are suitable for your situation. Not everything is relevant to you. You must pick what you think might be suitable and add it to what you already do. However, whatever you choose to do, follow the instructions to the letter.

It won't be long before your sense of self-belief returns; about three weeks of constant repetition of these techniques and hints is usually enough. Sometimes it can be as little as a week before you start to notice there's a changed attitude towards you.

Usually, you start to notice comments from others first, but you may start to feel more confidence after monitoring yourself in your diary. And your own sense of wellbeing, as you notice your improvement, is a key measure that your self-belief is rebuilding.

NOW, YOU "JUST DO IT"

Get into the habit of repeating the Nike running shoe mantra, Just do it. Rather than hum-ing and haa-ing over when and how to study.

Stop procrastinating and putting things off. Stop telling yourself, "I don't feel like it, I'll wait till I'm in the mood." Just do it. In other words, one way to set a habit is to just do it regardless of how you feel. Just make sure you're setting a good habit.

Colleagues will be more supportive and encouraging if you don't put study off. Consultants can get a bit disgruntled if they see you are not improving, you are not changing. You are the same person who's always been unsure and nervous.

It is better to make a mistake than to do nothing at all. We learn from our failures. How else do we learn? We don't learn from success. We learn from failure. An overseas-trained emergency medicine doctor I used to see, Ramish, had to sit the Australian Fellowship Exam so he could practise. He had already failed the written exams once, and he needed to pass to maintain his job. He was very reluctant to submit any of his written essays to colleagues to be evaluated. In fact, he had never asked anyone to look at his essays. He felt that his answers needed to be perfect, otherwise he would be embarrassed and humiliated. It was easier not to do anything. Also, he did not want to ask busy consultants to give up their precious time to mark his essays.

After some persuasion Ramish reluctantly agreed to ask consultants to mark his work. I pointed out to him that he should let the consultants know that he was doing the essays under strict exam conditions, so they would know he just wasn't trying to hand in the perfect answer. Ramish was pleasantly surprised by the reactions from consultants in his department. It wasn't what he had expected. They were keen to help him. They gave valuable advice, and Ramish was annoyed at himself that he hadn't asked for help sooner.

YOU DO IT REPEATEDLY

Let it come together through constant repetition, because repetition increases your ability to be fluent and articulate, and to respond clearly and get your message across. I worked with an oncology registrar who was initially reluctant to evaluate and monitor herself. Like most of us, she hated the sound of her voice, and cringed when she listened to herself. But she kept on practising recording and listening to herself, despite her reluctance. She noticed after a while it was easier to put her words together when responding to questions.

Okay, there will be days when you just don't do whatever it is you are supposed to be doing. That happens, and you shouldn't be too harsh on yourself. People do relapse occasionally, as we do with diets. We can be good about what we eat, and then all of a sudden, get a craving, sit down and demolish a large block of chocolate. Just take each day at a time and get back on the wagon the next day. Don't denigrate yourself and pull yourself down. Think, okay, that happened, and it just may happen again, but today I go back to my study routine. After all, it's not the pace and style that matters – slow and steady really will get me over the line.

OTHERS TREAT YOU DIFFERENTLY

A consultant nods, and says, "That was okay." A colleague says, "You sound more confident." Notice those compliments (however small). There's a cycle that occurs; the more self-belief you have and the more you follow these habits, the more people will give you positive feedback. The more positive feedback, the greater your self-belief and the easier it is to stick to your new study habits.

Ramish, the overseas-trained doctor I mentioned before, soon became aware that consultants were encouraging and praising more of his responses. The next time I saw Ramish, he was so delighted. He had just sat a full practice exam and had been told that he'd passed this easily. It certainly gave him a great deal of confidence for the next sitting of his Fellowship exam.

YOUR SELF-CONFIDENCE INCREASES WITH DAILY EVALUATION

Look at your diary. If you have followed my instructions, it will be full of notes and scores showing improvement. If you evaluate yourself daily, you get to know how you are going, and you'll see that the practice does improve your performance. This will increase your self-confidence.

Ramish's positive experiences led to a shift in his attitude towards the upcoming exam. He felt that he had a good chance of passing the exam. Previously, he felt downhearted, could see no way to improve, and felt concerned for his future.

This daily self-evaluation, this way of checking your good habits and making a change, is another cycle where you build your self-belief from the inside. You feel in control, you learn more in a shorter time frame and retain what you have learned, you become more fluent and articulate. This in turn, helps you also become more relaxed and connected to your family and friends.

YOUR NEGATIVE THOUGHTS HAVE DIMINISHED

A urology registrar I worked with told me how he used to panic if a consultant asked, "Are you sure?" or, "Is there anything more you want to say?" He thought he'd forgotten something. He would look at the consultant's face for some validation or approval, then he'd say something inappropriate or irrelevant because he couldn't stand the silence. He often had changed his response if he perceived the consultant's disapproval, sometimes changing a correct answer to an incorrect answer.

This was no longer happening. Now he was more confident about the correctness of his responses, he would take a breath, calm down and answer appropriately. When we reduce negative thoughts, we replace them with positive and constructive thoughts. Our whole attitude starts to change.

YOU WILL GET YOUR LIFE BACK

Life is not just study and work. Okay, in the last month or so before an exam, study will take a bigger part, but by then, you can see the light at the end of the tunnel.

I want to share with you an email I received from a doctor who sat for her exams four years ago after using the techniques that I have outlined in this book:

Dear Dr Tremayne,

I am so incredibly happy. My exam performance exceeded my expectations. I flew through the questions. It was undoubtedly the most intense three days so far of my life, but on reflection, I cannot believe how well I performed.

There were stations where I would manage to finish answering 40 verbal questions in the allotted six minutes and the exam planners would make up more questions for me because they are required to fill the allotted time.

This kind of success and self-belief can be yours if you want it to be. It is up to you.

As Stephen Covey once said "change – real change – comes from the inside out". How you respond to your experiences is what matters. You can make things happen through your initiative. If you, the reader of this book, have had the courage to change your study habits and have embraced regular testing of your knowledge, you have shown a capacity for change. Other changes will then take place. Your sense of security will improve. You will restore belief in your intrinsic value as a person. This will carry over to your relationships with family, your friends, and work colleagues. You have become more mentally tough. You have changed your reality.

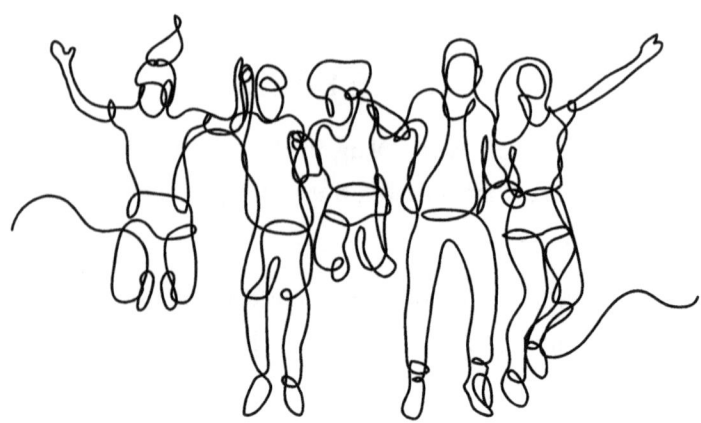

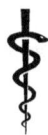

CONCLUSION

"Successful people aren't born that way. They become successful by establishing the habit of doing things unsuccessful people don't like to do."

WILLIAM MAKEPEACE THACKERAY

In performance psychology, we now understand that training our brain and our emotional responses is just an integral part of the high-performance environment. Doctors, like athletes, have a total commitment to the pursuit of excellence. When it comes to high performance, there is no question being mentally tough gives a medical trainee an advantage. Doctors have a need for psychological skills training and consequent mental toughness, to deal with the pressure, isolation, distractions, long hours at the hospital, the constant fatigue, and often the lack of motivation to be always studying for exams. Mental toughness is an attribute that some people already have. However, it can certainly be harnessed and developed through the regular practice of mental skill strategies in this book.

Mental or psychological skill strategies such as pre-performance routines, energy regulation, imagery, focusing and refocusing, and attentional control, are seldom utilised systematically by doctors. Mental skills training is used to help athletes develop the attributes of mental toughness, such as resilience, and the ability to perform under pressure. Why not use mental skills training for doctors and devise programs that build key areas essential to the training of doctors? When mental skill strategies are inserted consistently into the work and study environment, they can enhance the quality of performance, increase wellbeing, and lead to increased chances of success in examinations.

If doctors master the mental game, they are more likely to have a successful and meaningful career. Many of the techniques I teach are useful lifestyle skills people will carry with them forever.

I trust that the reading of this book has increased your awareness of your strengths and the areas that need improvement. The first three chapters remind you of the reality of being a medical trainee, the structure required for successful study, and how to recover from old study habits. In the second three chapters you learn more about attention and how it impacts your study, some evidence-based techniques, and testing under pressure conditions of the various exam components. In the final chapters, the importance of non-verbal communication to engage the listener is discussed: How habits are formed through repetition of practice; the elements of success; and then the increasing awareness of enhanced self-efficacy and self-belief as improvement takes place.

It is possible to develop a systematic individualised study program based on the readings in this book. Doctors who do this will have an increased capacity to move forward and get on with life. All the suggested techniques can be utilised, not only for study, but for other areas in life.

You can succeed and get that life back!

BIBLIOGRAPHY

Aarts, H. & Dijksterhuis,A.P. (2000). The automatic activation of goal directed behaviour: The case of travel habit. *Journal of Environmental Psychology, 20*, 75-82

Aubusson, K. (2019). *Exhausted surgeon dismissed. Sydney Morning Herald*, February 6, 12-13

Aubusson, K. (2019). *Doctors fight pressure to fudge hours. Sydney Morning Herald*, February 13, 3.

Bargh, J. & Chartrand, T.L. (1999). The unbearable automaticity of being. *American Psychologist, 54*(7), 462-479.

Baumeister, R.F., Bratslavsky, E., Muraven, M. & Tice, D.M. (1998). Ego depletion: Is the active self a limited resource? *Journal of Personality and Social Psychology. 74*, 1252-65.

Baumeister, R.F. & Scher, S.J. (1988). Self-defeating behavior patterns among normal individuals: Review and analysis of common self-destructive tendencies. *Psychological Bulletin, 104*, 3-22.

Beck, I. L., McKeown, M. G., & Kucan, L. (2002). *Bringing Words to Life*. Robust Vocabulary Instruction. New York: Guilford Press.

Beyondblue. (2013*). National mental health survey of doctors and medical students*. Melbourne: Beyondblue.

Blatter, K. & Cajochen, C. (2007). Circadian rhythms in cognitive performance: Methodological constraints, protocols, theoretical underpinnings. *Physiology & Behavior, 90*, 196-208.

Brown, K.W. & Ryan, R.M. (2003). The benefits of being present: Mindfulness and its role in psychological well-being. *Journal of Personality and Social Psychology, 84*, 822-848.

Chrysanthos, N. (2019*). Projects seek to address burnout among junior doctors. Sydney Morning Herald*, February 11.

Covey, S.R. (1989). *The 7 Habits of Highly Effective People*. London: Simon & Schuster.

Cuddy, A. (2016). *Presence: Bringing your Boldest Self to your Biggest Challenges*. London: Orion Publishers.

Doidge, N. (2007). *The Brain that Changes Itself: Stories of Personal Triumph from the Frontiers of Brain Science*. London: Penguin Books.

Epstein, M. (1995*). Thoughts Without A Thinker*. New York: Basic Books.

Epstein, M. (1998). *Going to Pieces without Falling Apart: A Buddhist Perspective on Wholeness*. New York: Broadway Books.

Fitts, P.M. & Posner M.I. (1967*). Human performance*. Belmont, CA: Brooks/Cole.

Haddad, K., & Tremayne, P. (2009). The effectiveness of centering on free throw shooting percentage with young athletes. *The Sport Psychologist, 1*, 118-136.

Hodges, B., Regehr, G., & Martin, D. (2001). Difficulties in recognizing one's own incompetence. Novice physicians who are unskilled and unaware of it. *Academic Medicine*, 76.

Kahneman, D. (2011). *Thinking Fast and Slow*. London: Penguin Books.

Kang, S.H.K. (2016). Spaced repetition promotes efficient and effective learning: Policy implications for instruction. *Behavioral and Brain Sciences, 3*, 12-19.

Kenny, D.T. (2011*). The Psychology of Music Performance Anxiety*. London: Oxford University Press.

Korotitsch, W., & Nelson-Gray, R. (1999). An overview of self-monitoring research in assessment and treatment. *Psychological Assessment, 11*, 415-425.

Marsh, H. (2017*). Admissions: A Life in Brain Surgery*. London: Weidenfeld & Nicholson.

Mehrabian, A. (1981). *Silent Messages: Implicit Communication of Emotions and Attitudes* (2nd Ed.). Belmont, CA: Wadsworth.

Morris, A., Spittle, M., & Watt, A. (2005). *Imagery in Sport*. USA: Human Kinetics.

Morgan, W. & Tremayne, P. (1985). *Measuring Up: Choosing an (almost!) painless diet and exercise plan*. Australia: Doubleday.

Navarro, J. (2008). *What Everybody is Saying: An Ex-FBI Agent's Guide to Speed-Reading People*. New York: Harper-Collins.

Newbery, G. & Tremayne, P. (2016). *Examining the efficacy of mental skills *training for the promotion of academic resilience in higher education.* Proceedings of the 14th Annual Hawaii International Conference on Arts and Humanities, Honolulu, Hawaii, [Digital Proceedings], (ISSN # 1541-5899), Jan. 9-12.

Orlick, T. (2000*). In Pursuit of Excellence: How to Win in Sport and Life through Mental Training.* (3rd Ed.). USA: Human Kinetics.

Prochaska, J.O. & DiClemente, C.C. (1984). *The transtheoretical approach: Crossing traditional boundaries of therapy.* Homewood, IL: Dow Jones-Irwin.

Restak, R. (2011). *Optimizing Brain Fitness.* Virginia, USA: The Great Courses.

Thayer, R. E. (1967). Measurement of activation through self-report. *Psychological Reports, 20,* 663-678.

Thayer, R. E. (1986). Activation-Deactivation Adjective Check List (AD ACL): Current overview and structural analysis. *Psychological Reports, 58,* 607-614.

Thayer, R. E. (1989). *The Biopsychology of Mood and Arousal.* NY: Oxford University Press.

Toastmasters International (2011). *Your Speaking Voice.* Retrieved 2018 from https://www.toastmasters.org/~/media/ B7D5C3F93FC3439589BCBF5DBF521132.ashx

Tremayne, P. & Ballinger, D. (2008). Performance enhancement for ballroom dancers: Psychological perspectives. *The Sport Psychologist, 22,* 90-108.

Tremayne, P. & Morgan, A. (2016). Attention, centering, and being mindful: Medical specialties to the performing arts. Invited chapter in A. Baltzell, (Ed.), *A Cambridge Companion to Mindfulness and Performance.* USA: Cambridge University Press.

Vealey, R., & Greenleaf, C.A. (2006). Seeing is believing: Understanding and using imagery in sport. In Jean M. Williams (Ed.). *Applied sport psychology: Personal growth to peak performance.* (5th Ed.). New York, N.Y.: McGraw Hill.

CPSIA information can be obtained
at www.ICGtesting.com
Printed in the USA
BVHW030838120822
644443BV00017B/346

9 780648 548201